Endoscopic Laser Surgery
of the Upper Aerodigestive Tract

To our Mentor
Malte Erik Wigand

Endoscopic Laser Surgery of the Upper Aerodigestive Tract

With Special Emphasis on Cancer Surgery

Wolfgang Steiner, M.D.

Professor and Chairman
Department of Otorhinolaryngology
and Head and Neck Surgery
University of Göttingen
Göttingen
Germany

Petra Ambrosch, M.D.

Associate Professor
Department of Otorhinolaryngology
and Head and Neck Surgery
University of Göttingen
Göttingen
Germany

With contributions by
Ulrich Braun, Wolfram Gorisch, and Eberhard Kruse

Translated by M.V. Knappe, edited by R.T. Gregor

298 illustrations

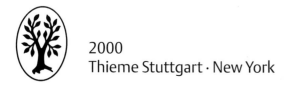

2000
Thieme Stuttgart · New York

Library of Congress Cataloging-in-Publication Data is available from the publisher.

Contributors' addresses:
Ulrich Braun, M. D.
Professor
Department of Anesthesiology and Intensive Care Medicine
University of Göttingen
Göttingen, Germany

Wolfram Gorisch, Ph. D.
Munich
Germany

Eberhard Kruse, M. D.
Professor and Chairman
Department of Speech Pathology and Pediatric Audiology
University of Göttingen
Göttingen, Germany

Translator:
M. V. Knappe, M. D., Munich

Translation editor:
R. T. Gregor, FRCS, Ph.D. FACS
Professor and Chairman
Department of Otorhinolaryngology
University of Stellenbosch
Tygerberg
Republic of South Africa

This book is an authorized translation of the German edition published and copyrighted 1997 by Georg Thieme Verlag, Stuttgart, Germany.

Cover drawing:
Renate Stockinger, Stuttgart

Important Note: Medicine is an ever-changing science undergoing continual development. Research and clinical experience are continually expanding our knowledge, in particular our knowledge of proper treatment and drug therapy. Insofar as this book mentions any dosage or application, readers may rest assured that the authors, editors, and publishers have made every effort to ensure that such references are in accordance with **the state of knowledge at the time of production of the book**.
Nevertheless this does not involve, imply, or express any guarantee or responsibility on the part of the publishers in respect of any dosage instructions and forms of application stated in the book. **Every user is requested to examine carefully** the manufacturers' leaflets accompanying each drug and to check, if necessary in consultation with a physician or specialist, whether the dosage schedules mentioned therein or the contraindications stated by the manufacturers differ from the statements made in the present book. Such examination is particularly important with drugs that are either rarely used or have been newly released on the market. **Every dosage schedule or every form of application used is entirely at the user's own risk and responsibility**. The authors and publishers request every user to report to the publishers any discrepancies or inaccuracies noticed.

© 2000 Georg Thieme Verlag,
Rüdigerstraße 14, D-70469 Stuttgart, Germany
Thieme New York, 333 Seventh Avenue,
New York, N.Y. 10001 U.S.A.

Typesetting by Mitterweger & Partner, Plankstadt

Printed in Germany by Staudigl, Donauwörth

ISBN 3-13-125271-5 (GTV)
ISBN 0-86577-996-1 (TNY)   1 2 3 4 5

Foreword

Wolfgang Steiner's und Petra Ambrosch's book is a major contribution to advance medical progress. Ever since he organized the first course on CO_2-laser surgery with me in 1979 at Professor Wigands's department in Germany, the surgical treatment of head and neck cancers changed in Germany. Continuing his work at the University of Göttingen, his workshops greatly contributed to a new concept and success of minimally invasive treatment of cancer.

In this "how to do" book detailed practical descriptions with excellent illustrations show that an important organ, the larynx, can be saved with relatively minimal trauma using laser surgery. It is well demonstrated that in a bloodless surgical field with higher magnification and with experience one can differentiate between normal and cancerous tissue. It is similar to seeing the difference in the pattern structure of an oriental rug. Experimentally placing small 25 micron diameter glass balls on a cut surface of cancerous tissue, one could estimate that with 25 times magnification a conglomerate of approximately 1-10 million cancer cells can be distinguished from normal tissue structure. Therefore, one can speak of microsurgery for cancer, which includes both diagnosis and treatment.

The book points out well that one can tailor the surgery according to the extension of cancer. If the cancer is localized in the endolarynx or in the hypopharynx, it is technically possible to eradicate it. For the necessary maximal exposure, special laryngoscopes and other instruments have been developed by the author. These are necessary to achieve the removal of cancer which should not be stopped until the experienced surgeon feels convinced at the end of the procedure that he removed everything visible through the microscope. Any shortcut will result in failure.

The necessary and well-described biopsy techniques are of utmost importance, as well as the recording of the position and tissue site. It is not unusual that one ends up with 10-18 specimens for the pathologist. The postoperative evaluation may also result in the need for additional tissue removal using the described minimally invasive microsurgical techniques.

Cutting through cancerous tissue to obtain specimens would be against the principles of conventional oncologic surgery. With microscopic laser surgery one can see the structure of the cut surface of the tumor. It is like cutting with a microtome under magnification; one can differentiate between malignant und nonmalignant structure. This way "the surgeon can individually adjust the safety margin."

When the cancer expands through the boundaries of the larynx into the cervical tissues a combined endolaryngeal and transcervical approach can be used. This way laryngectomy can be avoided. It is fortunate that glottic cancers cause early hoarseness and stay localized. If the patient gets early expert attention, a good functional voice and long-term cure can be achieved with laser surgery.

The book describes well how to treat cancer with minimally invasive laser surgery and how voice organs and other important structures can be preserved. The University of Göttingen has been in the forefront of these developments. The 20 years of experience, pioneering efforts, and enthusiastic work and workshops by Wolfgang Steiner and Petra Ambrosch contributed not only to a decrease in mortality but they also preserved the quality of life of many patients.

The global cancer statistics (Cancer Statistics, 1999, American Cancer Society) show that in 1999 there were 363,000 new cases of oral and pharyngeal cancers worldwide and 200,000 deaths. They also reveal that there were 135,000 new cases of laryngeal cancers and 73,500 deaths. This book describes the techniques and instrumentation which would be needed in oncologic centers around the world to decrease cancer mortality and to save tens of thousands of larynges yearly. This English publication will have a profound effect on worldwide medical progress.

Geza J. Jako, M.D.
Melrose (Boston), Massachusetts

Foreword

It is with great pleasure that I write these few words of preface to this important text developed by my dear friend and colleague, Wolfgang Steiner. He is indeed a master of transoral laser microsurgery who has truly pioneered a highly important area in the management of head and neck cancer.

The name Wolfgang Steiner is synonymous with endoscopic laser microsurgery of head and neck cancer. His name also calls forth the immediate recognitions of great enthusiasm, clearly defined opinions, and masterful surgery. While other surgeons have gained great expertise in transoral laser microsurgery, Steiner stands alone in his never deviating commitment to the benefits of this surgery. He clearly was one, if not the pioneer, of transoral laser microsurgery for laryngeal cancer. In an era where most other otolaryngologist-head and neck surgeons were highly skeptical of his technique, he continued with absolute commitment to an approach to conservative surgery that has benefited hundreds of patients.

Beyond Steiner's presence internationally, he has graciously hosted scores of head and neck surgeons in Göttingen so they could personally observe Wolfgang Steiner and Petra Ambrosch perform endoscopic laser surgery. These visitors have observed patients both in the perioperative period and long after their surgeries, and have then left Göttingen realizing they have experienced something very special which usually has transformed their vision of transoral laser microsurgery and clearly confirmed the validity of Steiner's work. More importantly, those trained by Steiner have learned key insights that have allowed them to more safely and effectively treat selected patients with this approach.

This book by Wolfgang Steiner and Petra Ambrosch is a thoughtful, clear, and extremely helpful guide to surgeons who desire to learn the basics of transoral laser microsurgery. The book is not a substitute for personal hands-on training under the direction of those who have gained expertise with this technique. On the other hand, this book provides many of the basic principles that will allow the thoughtful surgeon to effectively use this technique and benefit many patients.

When new approaches are presented to old problems, reactions vary remarkably from great excitement to outright condemnation by those often minimally familiar with what the new idea or approach truly represents. This statement certainly applies to the work of Wolfgang Steiner. It is now remarkably gratifying that many otolaryngologist-head and neck surgeons are seeing Steiner's work for what it really is: that of a masterful use of laser technology to perform conservation laryngeal and other head and neck cancer surgeries, following true oncological principles, and benefiting patients by the remarkably lower morbidity rate seen with this technique. Skeptics who feel transoral laser microsurgery violates basic oncological principles almost certainly need more insight into what is really being done by this approach. Wolfgang Steiner's work thoughtfully and carefully elucidates this core principle, which is essential to the true appreciation of what is presented here.

Those who thoughtfully and carefully study the chapters of this book will certainly be enriched in their understanding of transoral laser microsurgery and further facilitated in their ability to understand this work and apply it to the level that their training allows. I am personally most appreciative of Wolfgang Steiner, his freely shared insights, and his true friendship.

R. Kim Davis, M.D.
Professor and Chairman
University Medical Center
Salt Lake City, Utah

Foreword

Change is difficult. Change in medicine is usually evolutionary. Revolutionary changes in medicine that challenge long-held ideas require a strong belief in the new ideas and mass of data to support them. Wolfgang Steiner has championed the idea that many cancers of the larynx and other upper airway sites can be effectively treated transorally using the laser. He has accumulated the data to support the idea and has fearlessly exposed his work and his data to anyone willing to learn and consider change. In the process, a giant medical industry has been challenged.

The reality that some cancers of the larynx and laryngopharynx could be treated through the mouth is not a new one. Sporadic reports of transoral ablation of cancer have been written about since the early part of the 20th century. The idea was generally either unaccepted, unappreciated, or rejected as unsound. I recall the word "malpractice" used in a discussion of my paper on the endoscopic treatment of early cancer at the 1st Centennial Conference of Laryngeal Cancer held in Toronto. The idea that some cancers can be removed at the time of biopsy, an idea so simple and logical, was carried along by a few brave North American laryngologists, but a "more is better" attitude of the time prevailed in most North American centers. Endoscopic cancer surgery was generally unaccepted. The laser and the brillant illumination and magnification of the operating microscope made endoscopic surgery more attractive. It took the enthusiasm and resilience of Wolfgang Steiner and Petra Ambrosch to gather data and force our profession to reexamine some basic premises.

Cutting through cancer was anathema. Now cutting through tumor is a route to better exposure. Using the operating microscope as a guide to safe margins was unthinkable. Now it makes sense. Cutting through cartilage and deliberately operating with the laser in the pre-epiglottic space and neck was frightening. Now we can expand our boundaries with the knowledge that the pioneers were safely there before us. The knowledge and experience so willingly shared by Steiner and Ambrosch and so generously delivered to us in their book "Endoscopic Laser Surgery of the Upper Aerodigestive Tract" has set us free from principles that have shackled us to old ideas the were wrong for too long.

The timing of this new paradigm cannot be underestimated. For decades the North American surgeon worked with the principle that "more" and "bigger" was better. Then came cost containment, HMOs, minimally invasive surgery, outpatient surgery centers, and other mechanisms designed to limit health-care costs. "More" and "bigger" was no longer better. Cost-effective focused, efficient, and effective treatment was now better. In our specialty it was no longer acceptable to have lengthy hospital stays and major morbidity. With endoscopic laser surgery we have reduced treatment time for early glottic cancers from six weeks to one hour. Patients with supraglottic cancer treated endoscopically are out of the hospital in days rather than weeks. The quality of life issues of swallowing and voice are now being addressed in a reassuring way. We have made exciting progress.

To those who believe, no explanation is necessary, but the Steiner book delivers technical refinements and insights that will expand the surgeon's skill. To those who are skeptical, the book addresses, with data, the basic principles that will allow a beginning to what is, to me, a great adventure and probably the major positive change in head and neck oncology of the last three or four decades.

Lawrence W. DeSanto, M.D.
Professor Emeritus
Mayo Clinic Scottsdale
Rochester, Minnesota

Foreword

Cutting up large tumors and removing them through the mouth has generally been considered both unsound and impossible. However, if this actually could be done, it would fundamentally change the way we practice!

Wolfgang Steiner and Petra Ambrosch had a different vision. This book is the masters' work documenting this possibility for patients with laryngeal and pharyngeal cancer. I was privileged to attended a course they offered in 1996, expecting to learn what they were doing, so I could talk about it rationally at conferences. The sophistication of their techniques astonished me. As guests, we could sit down to their microscopes, make drawings, keep notes, and study the tools and techniques without hindrance.

At the end of the second day I began to consider actually introducing this technology into my practice. By the end of the third day, I felt an obligation to do so.

The concepts explained in this book deserve the careful attention of everyone who deals with head and neck cancer — particularly clinicians involved in the initial selection of therapy. Squamous cancers are more often cured by excision than any other single modality. But the risk and disability of open surgery often dissuades patients (and doctors) from choosing this option when it would do the most good. It is not the actual resection of the primary that hurts, but dismantling the neck and the laryngeal or mandibular framework to get to it. This book, and the monumental work upon which it is based, show how the natural passageways can be used.

Squamous cancers always start in these natural passageways, arising on an epithelial surface. Thus the laryngeal/pharyngeal lumen is the logical place to define the margins and commence a tailored resection. Suspension techniques bring the operating microscope into play. Open surgery may provide better access, but endoscopic surgery with the high magnification and illumination the microscope adds provides better visualization of healthy tissue versus cancer. There is no need to replicate the formal operation designed to encompass all cancers in that class. The surgeon can fit the resection to the cancer with a precision comparable to Mohs.

"Endoscopic Laser Surgery of the Upper Aerodigestive Tract" will take you well beyond the removal of small tumor specimens that can fit up the narrow lumen of a laryngoscope. By systematically subdividing larger tumors into five or six manageable pieces, Steiner and Ambrosch boldly overcome that barrier. They came into direct conflict with one of the most hallowed tenants in surgical oncology — the principle of "en bloc" resection. Halstead did not have a laser, however. If all cut surfaces are "seared" by the instrument that made them, viable tumor cell implantation is foiled at the source. And planned laser incisions that transect the primary cancer provide a huge bonus — intraoperative clarification of the third dimension, the exact depth of infiltration, which is crucial to a logical excision.

In my former practice (my own experince is now defined as pre- or post-Göttingen!), formal open resections such as hemilaryngectomy or supraglottic laryngectomy required ritual reconstructions to restore function. How could this be done through the mouth? Observing how unreconstructed tonsillectomy wounds generate new mucosa, the authors reasoned that secondary intention healing might be a benefit of laser excision. The strap muscles, framework, neighboring soft tissues, nerves, and blood vessels were intact. Thus recoveries (and shortened hospital stays) were a byproduct of this approach — reconstruction was simply obviated.

It is not unusual for a major technical advance, especially one that requires practitioners to retrain and retool, to be greeted with professional scepticism. At some point, however, and this book may well define this point for new enquirers, most of us attending the Göttingen course came to realize the true power of this important new technology and began a struggle to catch up. For me, that effort continues to this very day.

Transoral laser microresection is a mature technology now, thanks to the tireless dedication and creativity of Wolfgang Steiner, Petra Ambrosch, and their staff. It is arguably the optimal initial treatment for over half of the head and neck cancer patients we see. The authors have worked continuously for over 20 years to develop and teach the tools and techniques of this method. Their colossal contributions now move from their courses and scientific publications to a wonderful book, and in English too. US patients will be the primary beneficiaries, providing we manage the transition.

Bruce W. Pearson, MD
Professor and Chairman
Mayo Clinic, Jacksonville, Florida

Preface

In the treatment of benign and malignant disease of the upper aerodigestive tract, endoscopic and microscopic laser surgery is assuming a role of ever-increasing importance and widespread acceptance. Evidence in support of this fact is the continuous increase in the numbers of congresses, courses, and publications covering the various aspects of laser surgery.

Jako and Strong from Boston, United States, must be given credit for first introducing the CO_2 laser in microsurgery of the larynx in the early 1970s. I took my first steps in the field of laser surgery at the beginning of 1979, encouraged by my teacher Malte Erik Wigand. I remember with great gratitude Geza Jako standing by my side during my first laser procedures in Erlangen, Germany. Since then, a close friendship has developed between us.

The 1980s saw the laser becoming more established in the treatment of benign lesions in the larynx, particularly that of recurrent laryngeal papillomatosis. Testimony of this is found in the extensive literature dealing with this subject. By contrast, laser was only slowly incorporated into the treatment of malignancies, and this development was restricted to only a few centers throughout the world. Furthermore, the application of lasers was mostly limited to the excision of early vocal cord tumors. The first reports on successful use of laser in cancer surgery came from Strong and colleagues in Boston in 1975. Their guidelines regarding the indications of laser tumor surgery were subsequently followed almost religiously, with only few and limited alterations being made. Burian and Höfler were the first in Europe to successfully treat a glottic carcinoma with the laser. In the meantime, publications have appeared from more than 30 centers, mainly with respect to early laryngeal cancer. Considering the advantages of this treatment form and the good results that are achieved, it is surprising that the method has not found wider acceptance. It must, however, be mentioned that several centers have now started to employ the laser in the management of oral cavity and oropharynx tumors with a similar aim.

As early as the beginning of the 1980s, we expanded the indications for curative laser treatment at the Head and Neck Unit in Erlangen to include all regions and all tumor types. This was based on the excellent results that we had obtained with both the microsurgical laser resection of early tumors and with the palliation of very advanced or recurrent disease.

The interest in laser surgery and particularly its place in oncological therapy goes much further than the borders of our country. This has lead to great activity in the two centers in Erlangen and Göttingen, Germany, to fulfill the growing demands for congresses and publications. By combining our extensive patient material for purposes of documentation, analysis, and long-term follow-up, we were able to demonstrate the efficacy of our treatment concept.

Acknowledgments

It is at this point that we wish to express our gratitude to our teacher Malte Erik Wigand. He was a continuous source of encouragement and support during the conception and implementation of the new ideas. His faith in us was never broken, despite hefty criticism from the outside. The progress, which eventually found recognition with more and more colleagues, would not have been possible without his critical observations and control on the one hand and his optimistic and progressive nature on the other.

The growing publicity of the method and the achieved results lead to an increasing number of visiting colleagues showing interest in the technique. Since the beginning of the 1990s, we have regularly hosted laser courses in Göttingen. Demand for the manual supplied to the participants during this course has brought about the need for a more comprehensive book. To our delight, this wish, expressed by numerous individuals, could be fulfilled with the help of Thieme Publisher's, the lecturers at the courses, phoniatrician Eberhard Kruse, anesthesiologist Ulrich Braun, and physicist Wolfram Gorisch (Munich, Germany).

Finally, our special thanks are extended to Thieme Publisher's, who made the publication of this operative manual possible. In particular we would like to thank Dr. Clifford Bergman and Gert A. Krüger for the active role that they played in the realization of this project.

Göttingen, Summer 2000
Wolfgang Steiner and *Petra Ambrosch*

Contents

Introduction

The main emphasis of this book is on microsurgical laser treatment of malignant tumors in the upper aerodigestive tract. The possibilities and advantages of transoral laser surgery through the microscope are convincingly demonstrated in this context. This is of importance to any otorhinolaryngologist, not only at larger centers, who is increasingly confronted with patients suffering from a malignancy of the upper aerodigestive tract. These cases are encountered on an almost daily basis.

It is our intention to introduce the new management strategy, including surgical principles, based on our concepts, experience, and statistically analyzed data. Another motivation is to reconsider traditionally held views. Furthermore, practical details of diagnosis and surgical technique are described. On this basis, a textbook almost reminiscent of a "cookbook" has evolved. While the trainee is given an introduction, the more advanced surgeon is provided with subtleties and special aspects of the operative technique. In certain circumstances the book will be able to aid the surgeon in decision-making.

Topics such as appropriate anesthetic technique, use of special endoscopes and instruments for laser surgery, and technical aspects of lasers as well as laser safety have been included.

A separate chapter highlights the role of the speech pathologist in diagnosis, postoperative care, and rehabilitation of the patient. For benign and malignant disease, a detailed and extensive discourse of the surgical technique is given with detailed cover of the individual sites and pathologies. A large section has been reserved for laser treatment of carcinomas. With regard to this, special note has been made of the histological verification of the completeness of tumor resections. The limitations of the method are shown especially in the cases of advanced tumors. Some repetition has been unavoidable and has been deliberately left in place for purposes of emphasis. While some chapters cover general aspects, others focus in more depth on specific anatomical or technical issues.

At the end of the book the reader should be convinced that laser surgery is superior to conventional techniques in the treatment of certain diseases of the upper aerodigestive tract. This holds true particularly for the preservation of function, which is possible with this form of surgery compared to radical resections of parts of the anatomy. The reader should be able to follow step by step how this therapeutic goal is achieved and which factors play an important role in this process. Certainly surgical skills alone are not enough. It will become evident that there are a number of prerequisites for successful surgical treatment. A detailed knowledge of the endoscopic anatomy, experience in conventional surgery and microsurgery, and proficiency in the use of lasers are required, as is the ability to manage any major complication that might arise intraoperatively or postoperatively. The close liaison with the pathologist is of utmost importance. Finally, a good working relationship with the patient and detailed counseling guarantee the cooperation of the patient during therapy and the intensive and demanding aftercare.

The greatest danger for the patient is an inadequately experienced laser surgeon. Lack of oncological practice may lead to wrong indications, the limitations of the method may be disregarded, and unacceptable compromises made for the sake of preservation of organ or function. The responsible use of this new technique and the strict adherence to oncological principles for the benefit of the patient must always be the highest priority.

Both positive and negative experiences have been made in the past 20 years of laser surgery on more than 2800 patients with tumors of the upper aerodigestive tract. They should contribute to the successful implementation of laser surgery and prevent unnecessary disappointment for surgeons and patients.

The most pertinent textbooks and publications are listed under the references at the end of this book. This list is, however, restricted to those works and references that are of significance for the understanding of the book and for purposes of comparison with our own findings. The reader can find further references, which are more comprehensive, in the cited publications of our group.

1 Preparations for Surgery

Intubation, Jet Ventilation, and the Apneic Phase from a Laryngological Point of View

General anesthesia with endotracheal intubation is recommended for any surgery of the upper aerodigestive tract employing the CO_2 laser. Commonly a size 5 Mallinckrodt tube (inner diameter: 5 mm) is used, which causes little obstruction of the operative field. The cuff is filled with saline and protected with saline-soaked swabs. Further shielding of tube and mucosa is achieved by placing additional moistened swabs distal to the lesion to be operated on. Dyed swabs are preferable as they reduce light reflection and hence artifacts on the TV screen.

Infants and small children are usually intubated with an uncuffed Portex tube.

Advantages and Disadvantages of Jet Ventilation

The indications for jet ventilation were established during the 1970s, when this technique was extensively tested in our department. Today its use in laser surgery is limited mainly to subglottic lesions, especially stenoses, intubation and contact granulomas, and poorly accessible papillomas.

When jet ventilation is administered through a tube incorporated in the laryngoscope, an optimal position can not always be achieved. Another disadvantage is the passive movement of the vocal cords during ventilation. This precludes precise microsurgical operating. On the risks of semi-flexible or flexible ventilation catheters, see Chapter 4, p. 122. Because oxygen concentrations above 30% pose an increased risk of spontaneous ignition and combustion, most surgeons employing jet ventilation prefer to discontinue the ventilation while the laser is being used. This is termed operating in the "apneic phase."

Advantages of Endotracheal Intubation

Anesthetists have brought a number of arguments forward in favor of general anesthesia with endotracheal intubation, the most prominent being a safe airway allowing controlled ventilation and the prophylaxis of aspiration (see Chapter 4, p. 118ff.). From the surgical viewpoint endotracheal intubation offers the following advantages:

— Completely immobilized vocal folds due to the use of systemic muscle relaxants allow for microsurgery of high precision.
— Neither surgeon nor anesthetist are under any time constraints.
— Subglottic mucosa is protected by moistened swabs, which simultaneously shield the tube.
— During laser dissection of a lesion, which has been pulled medially with a grasping forceps (Fig. 1.**1a**), the danger of the laser beam accidentally hitting the subglottic or tracheal mucosa is avoided. In order to prevent accidental injury to distal mucosa during jet ventilation, a protective shield would have to be introduced, which prohibits grasping and medialization of tissue. Although the accidental impact of only few laser discharges on the distal mucosa bears no serious consequences, this can be avoided altogether by endotracheal intubation.
— Work in areas of difficult access within the larynx, such as the anterior commissure, requires frequent changes of the laryngoscope and manipulations such as pressure onto the laryngeal skeleton by an assistant. This calls for time and patience by surgeon and anesthetist. In the intubated patient, the time constraint is lessened.
— Advocates of jet ventilation often claim that lesions in the posterior larynx cannot be adequately accessed in an intubated patient. The use of a small tube and experience in microlaryngoscopic surgery, however, allow for precise resection of almost any lesion or scar tissue in the posterior larynx. By anteriorly displacing the tube with the tip of the small-sized laryngoscope, full access is gained to the interarytenoid area. This technique enables the surgeon to resect tumors with subglottic extension and even those with infiltration of the posterior cricoid cartilage, without having to sacrifice oncological principles.

Operating During Apneic Phase

Should the tube still obstruct the operative field, it can be removed after oxygenating the patient with 100% oxygen. When the oxygen saturation drops, the tube is safely reinserted via the operating laryngoscope. Performing the operation during this apneic phase is an excellent alternative to jet ventilation. Even repeated reintubation through the laryngoscope is preferable to long-term jet ventilation in these special situations, as, in our experience, it is deemed safer by both surgeons and anesthetists.

Instruments and Theatre Safety

Laryngo-Pharyngoscopes

The laryngoscopes designed by Kleinsasser and manufactured by Storz, Germany, have been modified to meet the requirements of laser surgery. A matt finish reduces light reflection, the integrated suction tubes are detachable, and smoke evacuation pipes are incorporated in the anterior blade of the laryngoscope. Different lengths and inner diameters are available (Fig. 1.**1b** and 1.**3**).

The following laryngoscopes have proved especially useful in daily practice:

- The closed laryngoscopes with narrow lumen and extra length, which is universally applicable in *children* and *adults* with *difficult access* to the endolarynx, where the medium-sized laryngoscope is inappropriate (often considerable pressure onto the larynx from the outside is necessary to gain adequate access to the inner larynx and especially the anterior commissure) (Fig. 1.**3b, c**), and for access to the inter-arytenoid area and the subglottis.
- The medium-sized, closed adult laryngoscope, which is used mainly for endolaryngeal work and in areas where the bivalved laryngoscope does not provide sufficient exposure (Fig. 1.**3a**).
- The distending laryngo-pharyngoscope for work on supraglottis and hypopharynx (Fig. 1.**4a**).

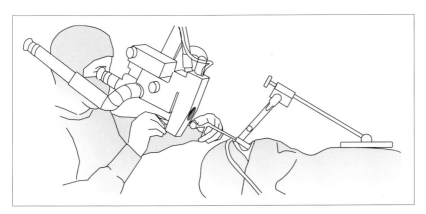

Fig. 1.**1a**   Drawing of the intra-operative situation during microlaryngoscopy with a CO_2 laser. The operating microscope is fitted with a 400 mm lens and micromanipulator control of the CO_2 laser beam. The laryngoscope has been introduced transorally and is supported on the platform above the patient's chest. The micromanipulator is manipulated by the surgeon's right hand, while the left is holding a grasping forceps introduced through the laryngoscope.

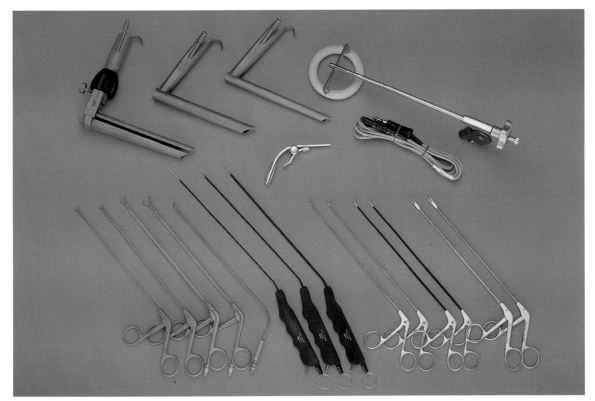

Fig. 1.**1b**   Basic laser microlaryngoscopy set.

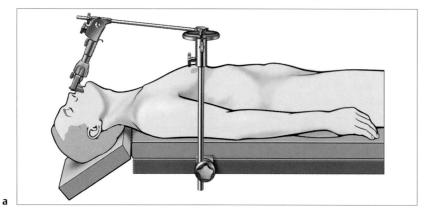

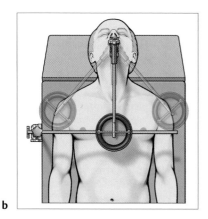

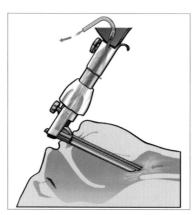

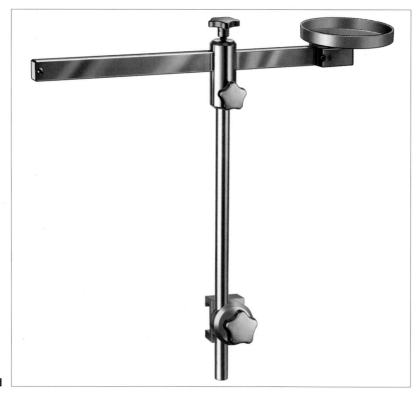

Fig. 1.2   Chest support with laryngopharyngoscope holder and supporting plate.
a Lateral view. b From above.
c Distending operating laryngopharyngoscope with integrated channel for evacuation of vapor.
d The adjustable supporting plate which can be secured in any three-dimensional position (b), allows effortless positioning of the laryngopharyngoscope during tumor surgery. Even extreme large angles are easily achieved and maintained.

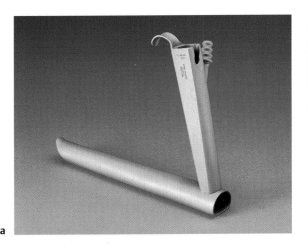

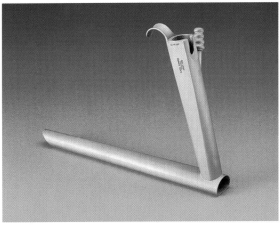

a

b

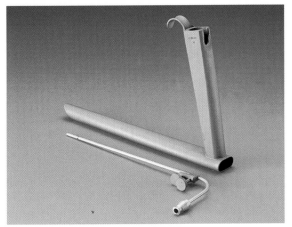

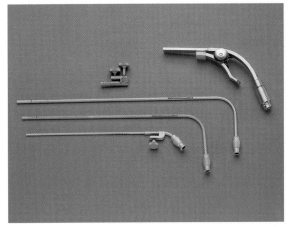

c

d

Fig. 1.3 Operating laryngoscopes with special matte finish and integrated suction channel for evacuation of vapor (**a, b**). **a** Medium-sized laryngoscope for routine procedures on the endolarynx (especially the glottic region). Due to its slightly upturned distal end this laryngoscope is suitable for exposure of the anterior commissure. **b** Small-sized, extra long (19 cm) laryngoscope for adults presenting with difficult exposure of the larynx (especially of the anterior glottis), for subglottic work; suitable for children. **c** Extra small-sized, long (20 cm) flat laryngoscope with attachable suction tube for difficult anatomical circumstances and children.

- The distending operating oropharyngoscope for procedures at tongue base, vallecula and lingual epiglottis. (Fig. 1.**4b**)

Advantages of the distending laryngopharyngoscope comprise a widely accessible operating field, improved orientation, and easier manipulation of instruments and better suitability for video documentation.

For operations on hypopharyngeal diverticula we use the diverticulum-scope by Weerda. Occasionally, the site of a tumor necessitates the use of a specially designed scope. These prototypes include a large-bore, extra-long adult laryngoscope as well as a small-bore, extra-long scope, with a slightly flattened cross section.

The laryngoscopes are supported by an adjustable platform, which is fixed to the operating table and has been specifically designed to meet the requirements of transoral laser surgery (Fig. 1.**2d**). Even the laryngoscope introduced from an almost lateral angle can be maintained in its position due to the wide range of possible adjustments.

Special Microinstruments

The development of laser-specific microinstruments was aimed at enabling the surgeon to operate effectively with a minimum number of instruments. Fig. 1.**5** and 1.**6** show the most important instruments in use.

Grasping forceps. Different designs of varying size with serrated or toothed jaws are being employed. They are used to gently hold small mucosal lesions or to forcefully retract larger pieces of tissue.

Suction tubes. Two well-insulated suction tubes of different inner diameter are useful not only for suction purposes and monopolar electrocautery but also as dissecting instruments and retractors of tissue during lasering, a function similar to that of a grasping forceps.

Coagulation forceps. For exact monopolar coagulation of small vessels or vascular stumps of small caliber protruding into the lumen, a microlaryngeal forceps with curved, serrated jaws is used. Bleeding from the

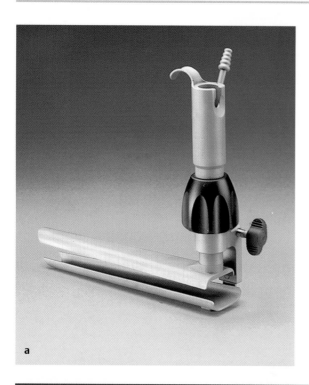

a

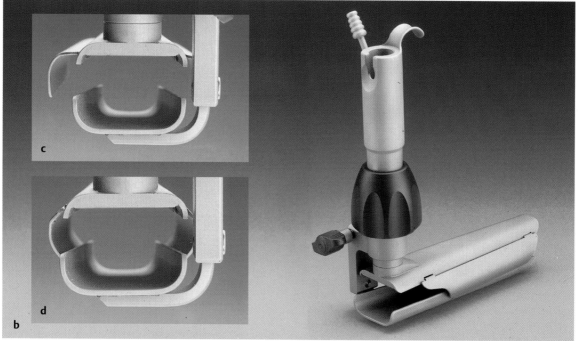

c

d

b

Fig. 1.**4**   Distending operating laryngopharyngoscope (**a**) and oropharyngoscope (**b-d**) with integrated suction channel for evacuation of vapor. **a** The distending operating laryngopharyngoscope is particularly useful for interventions in the hypopharynx and supraglottic region.

b Distending operating oropharyngoscope, suitable for laser-assisted surgery in the area of the base of the tongue. Bilaterally hinged blades prevent the tongue from obstructing the oropharyngoscope orifice. With integrated suction channel for evacuation of vapor. **c**, **d** Close-up view illustrating the nobility of the hinged blades.

Fig. 1.**5**   Microinstruments for transoral laser microsurgery, special matte finish, working length 22/23 cm.
a Grasping forceps, serrated jaws, alligator type, special matte finish. Available in different sizes, with or without suction channel for evacuation of vapor. **b** Grasping forceps, jaws curved right/left, serrated, insulated sheath.
c Grasping forceps, serrated, with triangular fenestrated jaws, curved upward left/right.
d Clip forceps, jaws curved left/right.

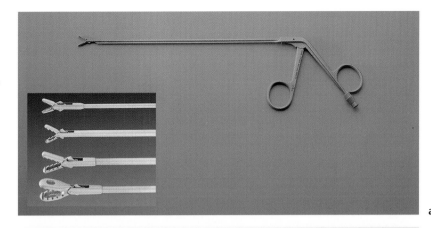

a

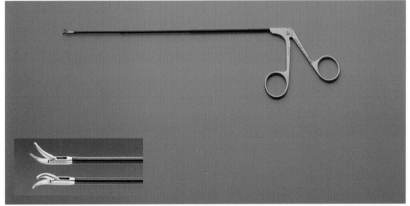

b

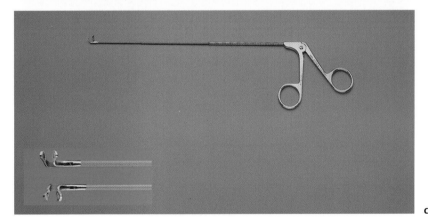

c

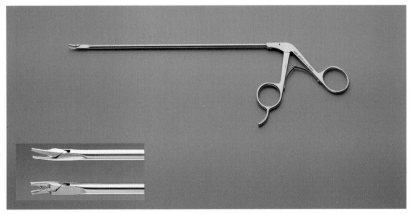

d

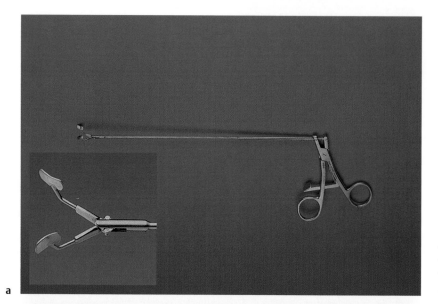

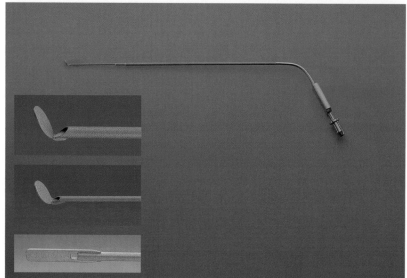

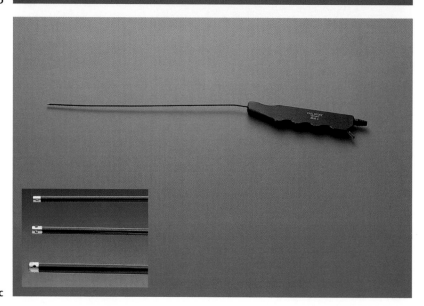

Fig. 1.**6** Micro-instruments for transoral laser microsurgery. **a** Retractor for visualization of the vocal cords retracting the false vocal cords and of the subglottis retracting the true vocal cords. **b** (top) Protector with suction channel for evacuation of vapor. Spatula shields the mucosa against accidental laser-beam exposure, for example, for protecting the glottis during laser surgery on the false vocal cord or for protecting the subglottis during laser resection of the free edge of the vocal cord in the unintubated patient. (buttom) Straight protector with suction tube. The distal elevator is suitable for protecting and retracting tissue. **c** Suction tubes different sizes insulated, for unipolar coagulation tubes. With ergonomic handle.

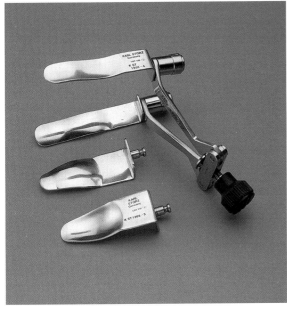
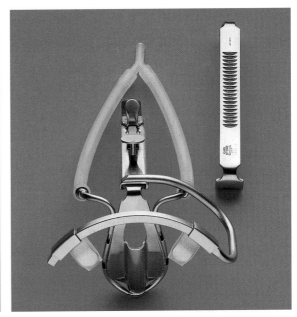

a   b

Fig. 1.**7**   Special retractors for oral cavity and oropharynx laser procedures. **a** Oral retractor set consisting of two adjustable arms with blades of different length and widths used to retract the cheeks for improved access to the oral cavity. **b** Oropharynx gag with groove for the endotracheal tube. Tongue depressor fitted with lateral openings and connectors on either side for the evacuation system.

cartilage, for example, can be controlled with this. Larger vessels, especially arteries (e.g., superior laryngeal or cricoid artery), are ligated using vascular *clips* (Fig. 1.**5d**).

Protecting shields. Different types of varying size and shape with incorporated suction tubes can be placed during laser surgery to protect the distal mucosa. Examples are: shielding of the subglottis during resection at the free edge of the vocal cord in the unintubated patient, protection of the vocal fold during operation on the false cord, or retraction of a healthy contralateral cord in patients with exophytic lesions of the anterior glottis (Fig. 3.**22**).

Special wide-angle Hopkins telescopes are indispensable for diagnosis, surgery, and postoperative treatment. Available in different directions of view, these telescopes are very useful for photo and video documentation in the upper aerodigestive tract. Other useful instruments include laser tracheobronchoscopes and the distending Weerda diverticuloscope. Benjamin laryngoscopes of different sizes are specially designed for laser surgery in neonates and children.*

Safety Precautions

The patient's face and particularly the eyes should be covered with a moistened green towel. The operating room staff must wear eye protection. Glass or plastic goggles are sufficient in the case of a CO_2 laser. This topic is dealt with in more depth in Chapter 6, p. 130ff.

Introducing the Laryngoscope

First a tooth guard is inserted. It is recommended that the right-handed surgeon introduce the laryngoscope from the right, with the endotracheal tube placed on the left (the position of the tube can be controlled digitally in the patient's pharynx). Care is taken to prevent the tongue from being caught between teeth and laryngoscope. When external pressure is required to visualize the anterior glottis, the laryngoscope must not be advanced beyond the level of the false cords. Cases with a small, floppy, Ω-shaped epiglottis can be problematic during introduction of the laryngoscope between endotracheal tube and epiglottis. The suprahyoid epiglottis may kink and the epiglottis double upon itself when it is "loaded" on the anterior blade of the laryngoscope. The trauma so caused can lead to postoperative edema and access to the anterior commissure made even more difficult.

> In these relatively rare cases a grasping forceps is useful to hold the epiglottis, while the laryngoscope is introduced with the other hand. Occasionally, a suture through the epiglottis is helpful to manipulate it from the outside.

---

* All laryngoscopes, laser microinstruments, and endoscopes are manufactured by KARL STORZ, Tuttlingen, Germany

Cutting Technique

Modern laser technology allows working with a focused laser beam and cuts almost without carbonization. The micromanipulator control, which is predominantly used in our department, gives a focus of 0.5 mm diameter. With the laser set at 6 W, one therefore operates at 3056 W/cm^2; with a setting of 20 W, at 10 188 W/cm^2.

When cutting through soft tissue, it is advantageous to follow a fine zigzag line with the toggle stick. Due to the physical characteristics of the laser, both its cutting and coagulating properties are thereby used to their maximum advantage. During laser dissection, it is recommended to repeatedly remove any char forming on the cut surface, by wiping it with a moist swab.

> To achieve hemostasis, the use of swabs or neuro "patties" can be helpful to compress feeding vessels. With the nondominant hand, the suction cannula (Fig. 1.**6c**) is pressed onto the swab to compress the vessel(s), with the other hand a grasping forceps for coagulation (Fig. 1.**5b**) is used to effectively stop bleeding.

Video Demonstration and Video Documentation

This enables anesthesiologist and operating room staff as well as surgeons in training or visitors to follow the operation on the screen. It provides for faster and more effective cooperation with the scrub sister. In case of a hemorrhage, for example, an experienced nurse will be able to act swiftly and appropriately.

A further advantage is the objective documentation of preoperative, intraoperative, and postoperative findings, or the continuous recording of the operation for teaching purposes.

Video documentation of important steps during surgery is extremely helpful for a retrospective analysis correlating the intraoperative clinical aspects with the postoperative histological findings.

Counseling for Laser Operations

The preoperative consultation with the patient must include counseling for microlaryngoscopy and panendoscopy.

Laser-specific risks. Only the extremely rare ignition of the tube constitutes an immediate danger from the use of a laser. This may lead to mucosal burns and in extreme cases can result in a secondary stenosis, or even necessitate a tracheotomy. One such case occurred at our department in the early days (1979), when air was used to inflate the cuff and no further protection employed. Fortunately this had no consequences for the patient, and no tracheotomy was necessary. When the appropriate safety measures are adhered to (saline to inflate the cuff, shielding of the tube, operating in the apneic phase in certain situations), this risk is so low that it is not included in the routine counseling of our patients. Over the last 20 years we have made routine use of the Mallinckrodt MLT tube, which is not specifically designed for laser surgery.

Complications. The counseling of our tumor patients focuses mainly on complications arising from the extent of the resection, such as *secondary hemorrhages* or *airway compromise* requiring reintubation or very rarely a tracheotomy. Wound healing is slightly protracted compared to conventional wounds. Before procedures on the vocal cords, patients are informed about postoperative hoarseness and voice rest is prescribed (Chapter 5, p. 125ff).

Furthermore, the patient is counseled about the possibility of persisting granulation tissue that requires repeated ablation for months after the surgery, and the development of webs and stenoses after extensive resections. Symptomatic mucosal edema, for example, in the area of the arytenoid cartilage after partial laryngectomy, may require postoperative administration of corticosteroids or rarely a laser excision of the edematous mucosa.

The oncological aspects are also discussed with the patient during the preoperative consultation. For example, the individual resection margin of an operation on the vocal folds is included in the counseling. A number of different factors, such as the patient's occupation, age, and the individual's need for oncologic safety are thereby taken into consideration. The patient must be aware that positive margins confirmed by the final histological report may be an indication for further resection. Finally, the patient needs to be informed about the possibility of local recurrence and second primary tumors, and the resulting need for a close and thorough follow-up. This surgical aftercare, especially during the first two years postoperatively, must be emphasized in particular.

2 Endoscopic Microsurgical Laser Treatment of Benign Diseases of the Upper Aerodigestive Tract

Intranasal, Transnasal, and Transoral Laser Microsurgery

Benign Diseases of the Nose, Paranasal Sinuses, Nasopharynx, Anterior Skull Base, and Orbit

Indications:
- Cauterization for epistaxis (including Osler–Weber–Rendu disease),
- Reduction of hypertrophied turbinates (Fig 2.**1**),
- Resection of septal spurs,
- Removal of benign tumors such as polyps, cysts, and papillomas
- Resection of vascular lesions such as angiofibromas and hemangiomas,
- Resection of postoperative granulation tissue, edema, recurrent or residual polyps, and synechiae,
- Resection of stenoses and scars in nasal cavity, lacrimal ducts, and nasopharynx,
- Opening of choanal atresia,
- Removal of residual adenoidal tissue.

Diagnosis: Routine transnasal and transoral endoscopy is performed with either rigid or flexible endoscopes. Computed tomography (CT) images must be obtained in cases of nasal polyposis, stenosis, and choanal atresia.

Type of laser: Argon or Nd:YAG laser, CO_2 laser.

Surgical technique: The procedure is performed endonasally under visual control (either through the 0° or 25° endoscope or through the microscope). General or local anesthesia can be used.

Choanal Atresia

The laser resection of congenital nasal cysts causing obstruction is comparatively easy. However, the surgery for choanal atresia, especially bilateral cases in the newborn, can be fraught with difficulties.

During recent years the microscope and CO_2 laser have become our preferred instruments.

Operative Procedure

A moistened gauze swab is introduced into the nasopharynx in order to protect the mucosa. It is removed in regular intervals throughout the operation to monitor the area transorally with a 70° telescope, or sometimes preferably a 90° telescope.

- During the procedure, special care should be taken not to work too far laterally. This is a high-risk area due to the proximity of the internal carotid artery.

Medially, i.e., adjacent to the vomer, tissue may be removed with greater impunity. The same applies to the area along the floor of the nose. At the end of the procedure, the wound is wiped with a wet gauze swab to remove any residual char which might induce the formation of granulation tissue.

Perioperative measures. In the 1980s, we regularly inserted stents in the form of silicone tubes to prevent re-stenosis. However, during the past few years we have moved away from this toward leaving the wound open. This is only possible if an opening can be created that anatomically resembles a natural choana.

Postoperative measures. Parents are instructed to suction the nose of their child with a thin catheter and regularly instill nasal ointment. In weekly intervals, the area is inspected by the otolaryngologist with a thin, rigid or flexible endoscope. In cases with a marked tendency toward formation of granulation tissue, the laser procedure should be repeated as early as possible.

Benign Neoplasms

The localization and extent of *vascular tumors*, such as angiofibromas and hemangiomas, determine whether they can be completely resected by laser alone. Often additional coagulation with conventional methods is necessary. The use of the CO_2 laser is limited in extensive, highly vascular neoplasms. The Nd:YAG laser is more useful in vascular lesions where coagulation is needed.

Hyperplastic changes of the nasal mucosa (septum, turbinates) as well as (isolated) *polyps* are theoretically amenable to laser resection, the Nd:YAG laser being the more appropriate choice due to its superior coagulating properties. However, the application of laser in these cases is slightly more demanding in terms of time and equipment, although it has the distinct advantage of markedly reduced intraoperative bleeding. Often limited surgery can be performed on an ambulatory basis, without the requirement for any nasal packing.

Laser for lesions in the nose is not widely used, mainly because of high equipment costs, but also due to its greater technical demands and prolonged operating time. Scherer from Berlin, Germany, is convinced, however, that this laser technique for nose and paranasal sinuses will find widespread approval in the rhinological practice of the future.

The Nd:YAG laser has the additional advantage that applications can be extended to work within the paranasal sinuses via flexible fibers which allow the resection (marsupialization) of *maxillary sinus* cysts via a

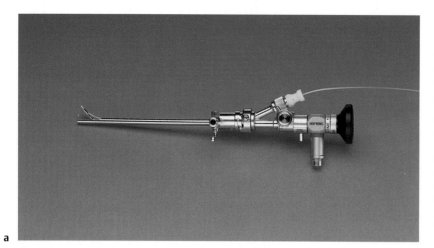

a

Fig. 2.1   Laser treatment of the inferior turbinate. **a** Laser rhinoscope with 30° telescope and Nd:YAG laser probe inserted into the working channel. **b** Distal tip of the rhinoscope sheath with deflecting device to guide the laser fiber. **c** Rhinoscope with a laser fiber in operating position within inferior nasal meatus. **d** Laser contact treatment of the inferior turbinate leaves a slightly carbonized, slit-like wound. **e** Some weeks after laser treatment; the turbinate is reduced in size and a scar is visible in the area of the surgery.

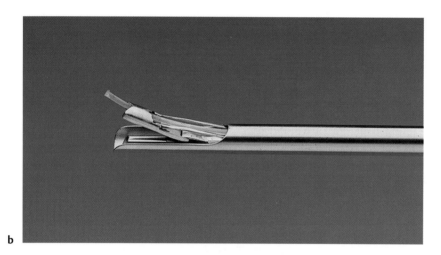

b

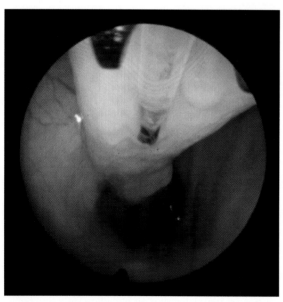

c

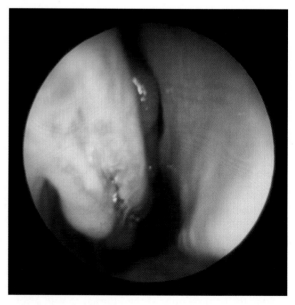

d

middle meatus antrostomy. Excessive *granulation* tissue forming postoperatively or recurrent polyps in the paranasal sinuses can be vaporized. Finally, the Nd:YAG laser is suitable for the *coagulation of small vessels*, for example, in Osler's disease, but of limited use in more severe hemorrhages.

An argon or Nd:YAG laser can be employed in the nasopharynx, under visual control of endoscopes, which can be inserted transnasally or transorally. Adenoidal tissue, cysts, and other benign lesions can be vaporized; scar bands forming between the roof of the nasopharynx and the Eustachian tube orifice after adenoidectomy can be divided. In our opinion, however, these laser procedures are only rarely indicated.

Benign Diseases of the Trachea

Indications:
— Pediatric patients: papillomas, granulation tissue, and stenoses after long-term intubation.
— Adult patients: stenoses secondary to endotracheal intubation and tracheotomy, fibromas, chondromas.

Diagnosis: Routine endoscopy is performed either under general anesthetic at microlaryngoscopy, or under topical anesthetic with the flexible endoscope. In certain cases imaging techniques are needed, preferably CT scans.
Type of laser: Nd:YAG, argon, and CO_2 laser.
Surgical technique: The laser treatment is administered through the rigid bronchoscope with a ventilator connection or through the supported laryngoscope in apnea or during jet ventilation.

Operative Procedure

The patient is ventilated with a mask. After administration of a short-acting muscle relaxant, the laryngoscope is introduced and supported on the platform above the

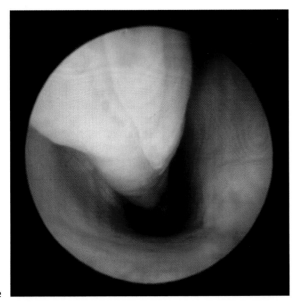

e

patient's chest. A 25° telescope is inserted through the laryngoscope, the trachea inspected, and the findings documented.

After intubation through the laryngoscope, the patient is ventilated with pure oxygen. The endotracheal tube is removed for the ensuing laser treatment. During the apneic phase, the argon or Nd:YAG laser can be used to resect the papilloma, the fibroma (Fig 2.**2**), or the scar stenosis under vision.

Of the tracheal stenoses, the membranous, sickle-shaped variety is best suited for this form of therapy (Fig 2.**3**). Single or repeated laser treatment can have long-term success. In more extensive stenoses with circumferential or lengthy scar formations, laser treatment alone is rarely sufficient. Some tracheal stenoses are caused by an inflammatory reaction and subsequent shrinkage of the tracheal cartilages, which is best appreciated radiologically. In these cases conventional surgical techniques should be employed.

Instead of operating in an apneic phase, the procedures can be performed during jet ventilation. For this purpose, a thin ventilating tube is placed distal to the stenosis.

The patient must be fully and continuously relaxed to avoid excessive pressure in the lungs, which may result in pneumothorax.

While the laser beam is applied to the tissues, the oxygen concentration should not exceed 30%.

Intraoral and Transoral Laser Microsurgery for Benign Neoplasms

Benign Diseases of the Oral Cavity and Oropharynx (Tonsils, Palate)

Indications:
– Papillomas, fibromas, granulomas, cysts, ranula,
– Hemangiomas,
– Leukoplakia, erythroplakia,
– Hyperplasia of gingiva (secondary to ill-fitting dentures),
– Lymphatic hypertrophy of ring of Waldeyer:
  • Hypertrophic tissue in lateral pharyngeal wall
  • Extensive granular pharyngitis, resistant to therapy
  • Tonsil hypertrophy in children (indications for partial laser tonsillectomy are controversial)
  • Chronic tonsillitis (tonsillectomy)
– Snoring (partial resection of soft palate).

Diagnosis: Inspection of the oral cavity and oropharynx, if necessary through the microscope. In certain cases a smear for cytological examination may be taken of lesions suspicious of malignancy or premalignancy. Rarely is a primary biopsy indicated. Angiography or magnetic resonance imaging (MRI) must be considered in vascular tumors.
Type of laser: CO_2 laser.
Surgical technique: The surgery is performed by intraoral or transoral microsurgical laser resection.

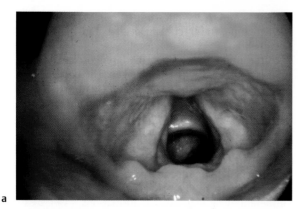

a

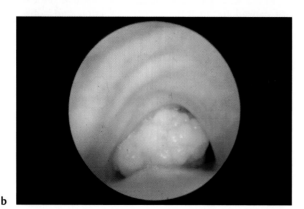

b

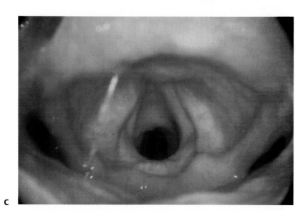

c

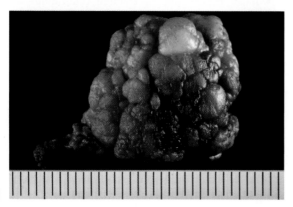

d

Fig. 2.**2**   Tracheal fibroma before, during, and after endoscopic resection with an argon laser. **a** At endoscopic view (90° telescope) a yellowish tumor is noticeable distal to the cricoid cartilage; it caused the patient severe dyspnea. **b** Intraoperative finding; the exophytic tumor takes its origin from the posterior tracheal wall and has almost completely obstructed the trachea. **c** View through the telescope after laser resection of the fibroma. **d** Surgical specimen.

Special oral retractors and an oropharynx gag with integrated evacuation system for vapor improve exposure (Fig. 1.**7**).

Operative Procedure

All lesions mentioned above are resected using the CO_2 laser under microscopic control and are examined histologically. Small lesions can be operated on under local or topical anesthetic on an outpatient basis. Hemostasis is generally not required for these superficial excisions. The patients suffer little or no pain and the wounds heal without significant scarring, making the site of excision almost invisible after healing. Larger hemangiomas usually require additional hemostasis by conventional methods. The Nd:YAG laser is recommended for highly vascular lesions.

Laser Operations on the Ring of Waldeyer

Treatment with the CO_2 laser is an alternative to the various forms of electrocautery for the management of extensive lymphatic hyperplasia of the posterior pharyngeal wall (severe granular pharyngitis, recurrent pharyngitis after tonsillectomy).

Tonsillar Hypertrophy in Children

During the last few years some authors (Scherer, 1994) have advocated partial laser ablation of tonsils (tonsillotomy according to the recommendations of Jako [Boston]) for the treatment of severely hypertrophied tonsils in children. This is recommended as an alternative to unilateral tonsillectomy in cases presenting as upper airway obstruction without the stigmata of chronic tonsillitis.

Chronic tonsillitis. In the routine treatment of chronic tonsillitis with or without tonsillar hypertrophy and peritonsillar abscesses we prefer *conventional* tonsillectomy. In the hands of an experienced surgeon the tonsil is usually removed quickly, completely, and with little blood loss. There is much less expenditure in terms of apparatus and time compared to laser tonsillectomy. Despite some advantages, the laser will not become established as an instrument for routine tonsillectomies. The use of the laser for a tonsillectomy becomes an obvious choice, however, when one is working with the laser on a daily basis and prefers a dry operating field under the microscope. It is also a useful method in patients with known clotting abnormalities (e.g., hemophilia). In cases of suspected cancer the laser has an

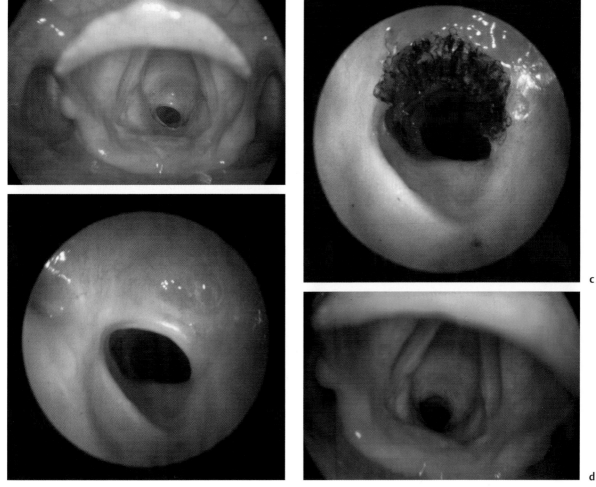

Fig. 2.**3** Tracheal stenosis after intubation before, during, and after endoscopic resection with an argon laser. These membranous stenoses have a relatively good prognosis with single or repeated laser treatment. In cases of extensive stenoses single modality laser treatment (CO_2, Nd:YAG, or argon) is usually not sufficient. **a** Endoscopic view (90° telescope) of the web-like scar in the anterior and posterior trachea. **b** Intraoperative findings. **c** Immediately after ablation of the anterior web with an argon laser. **d** Endoscopic view after single treatment with an argon laser.

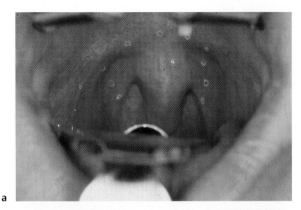

a

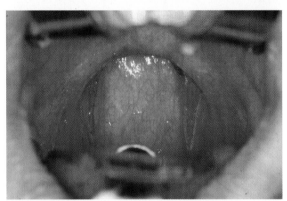

b

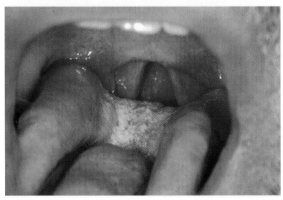

c

Fig. 2.**4** Partial resection of soft palate with an CO_2 laser for snoring. **a** An enlarged uvula and a flaccid soft palate are seen. The lines of resection are marked at the beginning of the operation. **b** The defect after resection of the uvula, parts of the soft palate, and the tonsillar pillars at the end of the procedure. **c** Eight weeks postoperatively scar formation has resulted in a tightened soft palate without affecting speech or swallowing function. The 60-year-old patient underwent simultaneous bilateral reduction of hypertrophied inferior turbinates. His headaches, the snoring, and his impaired nasal breathing were gone postoperatively.

advantage as a excision biopsy instrument because of the sealing effect (Werner, 1993). We use this routinely to perform biopsies during the examination of a patient with a neck mass and an occult primary. (For tonsillectomy and wedge-resection of the tongue base).

Advantages: Precise dissection with minimal hemorrhage is made possible. Optimal preservation of tonsillar pillars and pharyngeal musculature is achieved. A smaller wound, less blood loss (due to laser incision and immediate conventional cauterization with, for example, bipolar diathermy forceps) and less pain in the first postoperative days are the results.

Disadvantages: The procedure is more time-consuming, technically more difficult, and requires expensive equipment. Wound healing is slightly prolonged.

Finding the correct plane of dissection around the tonsillar capsule at the superior pole can be difficult. After the incision with the laser, spreading the tissues with scissors can be helpful in defining the capsule. We perform the operation with the patient's head in hyperextension, resulting in a tangentially incident laser beam on the mucosa. In some patients this would lead to excessive resection of mucosa at the superior pole if one uses the laser alone. Vaughan from Boston, United States, preserves the tonsillar capsule during laser operations by first resecting the bulk of the tonsil with the CO_2 laser and then vaporizing the remnants. Apparently, fewer postoperative hemorrhages and less pain are the advantage.

Partial Microsurgical Laser Resection of the Soft Palate for Snoring

Indications

A general physical and otorhinolaryngoscopical examination are essential to determine these. A hypertrophic uvula and/or atonic soft palate are commonly found. We generally perform a laser resection of a small part of the soft palate, including the uvula, and often combine this with a procedure aimed at improving the nasal airway. In our experience this procedure can be performed quite easily without a simultaneous tonsillectomy.

Operative Procedure

We commence the partial resection of the soft palate approximately 5 mm superior to the base of the uvula, using a CO_2 laser. The resection continues laterally into the tonsils, if they are to be preserved, and includes the cranial parts of the tonsillar pillars (Fig. 2.**4**). We do not insert any stitches for better approximation of the wound. During the first few postoperative days the patients usually have some difficulties swallowing fluids, with some escape through the nose. None of our patients, however, has suffered any permanent swallowing or speech problems.

We often use the combined approach of improving the nasal airway and simultaneously partially resecting soft palate and uvula. With the correct indications, this achieves a satisfactory result for the patient in over 90% of cases.

Benign Diseases of the Oropharynx (Tongue Base, Vallecula)

Indications: Hyperplasia of the tongue base, cyst, papilloma, hemangioma, lymphangioma, and others.

Diagnosis: Microlaryngoscopy is performed. Imaging techniques might be necessary in selected cases. In the case of suspected ectopic thyroid tissue a radionuclide study should be obtained.

Type of Laser: Preferably CO_2 laser.

Surgical technique: The surgery is performed via transoral approach and a microsurgical technique is used. The laser resection is done through the distending oropharyngoscope (Fig. 1.**4b-d**).

Operative Procedure

Large lesions require blockwise resection. This technique allows better visualization of the operative field and therefore provides for improved preservation of normal tissue.

Congenital benign lesions of the upper digestive tract can result in a compromised airway. The primary aim of endoscopic laser surgery is to alleviate the airway obstruction and thus prevent a tracheotomy. Large cysts of the tongue base can cause significant respiratory distress at birth. An aspiration of the cyst can be performed by the pediatrician in the intensive care unit in order to empty the cyst, lessen the obstruction, and facilitate an intubation. Soon afterward, however, a laryngologist should carry out a definitive endoscopic resection or marsupialization. In cases of hemangiomas an initial "wait and see" policy should be adopted. Only severe functional impairments, such as respiratory distress or aspiration, require active endoscopic surgical management.

In the adult, cysts or papillomas only rarely require laser surgical treatment. They are either accidental findings or the lesions are so large that symptoms such as globus or foreign body sensation are caused. Rarely does bleeding from the area around the vallecula require endoscopic (laser) coagulation.

Hyperlasia of the Tongue Base

In cases of well-circumscribed hyperplasia in the area of the tongue base, ectopic thyroid tissue and malignant lesions such as lymphoma or squamous cell carcinoma must be ruled out. Marked hyperplasia of the base of tongue can result in swallowing problems, globus sensation, and halitosis. Recurrent infections (lingual tonsillitis) may present as temperature spikes of unknown cause and odynophagia similar to tonsillitis. In these cases it is recommendable to surgically remove the chronically inflamed, hyperplastic lingual tonsil with the laser.

Operative Procedure

In this operation it is important to gain access to the tongue base through the distending oropharyngoscope (1.**4 b-d**) in such a way that the transition from normal tongue base to hyperplasia becomes clearly visible. The aim is to restrict the operation to the ablation of the hypertrophic lingual tonsil. If the resection remains within the lymphoid tissue without exposing tongue musculature, the intraoperative bleeding is limited and the patients have significantly less postoperative pain and odynophagia.

> Poor exposure can lead to difficulties during the resection, even if the principle of "as much as necessary and as little as possible" is followed. Laser procedures in the area of the tongue base are among the most difficult with regard to the surgical technique

> In cases of extensive hyperplasia and difficult access, removal of the oropharyngoscope at regular intervals is recommended. It is then possible to palpate the region or introduce the McIntosh laryngoscope in order to inspect the area of the tongue base either directly or through a telescope. Sometimes exposure with a gag as used for tonsillectomy is helpful.

Perioperative measures: Patients undergoing very extensive resections are given perioperative antibiotic prophylaxis. A nasogastric tube is usually not necessary. During the first postoperative days, a fluid diet is recommended. Analgesics are usually required. One of our patients, however, suffered from severe neuralgia in the distribution of the glossopharyngeal nerve for some weeks following the surgery.

Laser Surgery for Benign Diseases of the Hypopharynx

Indications: Cysts, papillomas, hemangiomas, diverticulae, cricopharyngeal achalasia (endoscopic laser myotomy).

In general, a laser surgical intervention is rarely indicated for benign lesions, since they are mostly discovered accidentally and hardly ever cause any symptoms. There are, thus, no strict criteria for an operation. Surgery should be contemplated depending on localization, extent, symptoms, and progression of disease.

Diagnosis: Clearly benign lesions, for example, cyst, edema, papilloma, etc. require only endoscopy (diagnostic and therapeutic in one session). *Vascular lesions,* for example hemangioma, may need angiography to assess vascular supply and extent of the tumor. In cases presenting with a *non-specific prominence* especially of posterior and/or lateral hypopharyngeal wall and tumors with smooth surfaces, differential diagnoses are: Forestier's disease, thyroid gland, lymphoma, metastasis, squamous cell carcinoma, and others. Additional radionuclide studies, radiological investigations, for example, lateral neck radiograph, CT, or MRI might be indicated. Certain lesions require a biopsy. If a

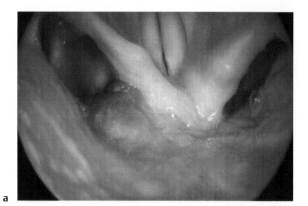

a

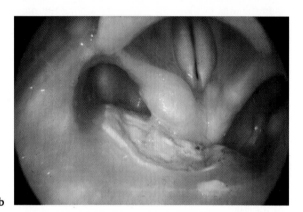

b

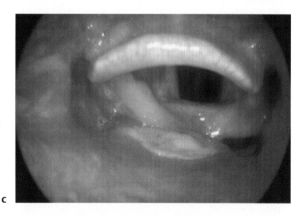

c

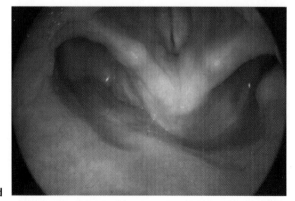

d

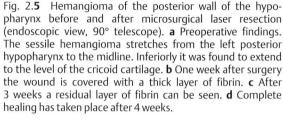

Fig. 2.**5** Hemangioma of the posterior wall of the hypopharynx before and after microsurgical laser resection (endoscopic view, 90° telescope). **a** Preoperative findings. The sessile hemangioma stretches from the left posterior hypopharynx to the midline. Inferiorly it was found to extend to the level of the cricoid cartilage. **b** One week after surgery the wound is covered with a thick layer of fibrin. **c** After 3 weeks a residual layer of fibrin can be seen. **d** Complete healing has taken place after 4 weeks.

Zenker's diverticulum is suspected, a Barium swallow (Fig. 2.**7a**) and endoscopy (diagnostic-therapeutic) should be performed.

Type of laser: CO_2 laser. For the treatment of hemangiomas (Fig. 2.**5**) perhaps combined with a Nd:YAG laser.

Operative procedure: Laser surgery is performed transorally under the microscope through the distended laryngopharyngoscope. The procedure depends on the findings. For example, a small cyst is excised; a large cyst is marsupialized. Clearly benign lesions (papillomas) are excised, larger tumors of unknown pathology are treated by primary incisional biopsy using the laser and immediate examination by frozen section.

Zenker's Diverticulum

Aim of the operation: Transmucosal cricopharyngeal myotomy.

Principle of the operation: The septum between upper esophagus and diverticulum is transected in the midline. This contains the upper esophageal sphincter in its superior portion. A large lumen combining diverticulum and esophagus is created and provides a wide passage for the swallowed food.

Type of laser: CO_2 laser.

Surgical technique: The operation is performed transorally, through a diverticulum scope (Weerda) under microscopic control. General anesthesia is given and the patient is positioned as for microlaryngoscopy with the head in hyperextension.

Operative Procedure

Esophagoscopy is performed (with telescopes) and the diverticulum inspected (to rule out a malignancy). The bivalved diverticulum scope is inserted with the longer upper blade in the esophagus and the slightly shorter one in the fundus of the diverticulum. The blades are then carefully opened to expose the muscular septum, which is brought under tension (Fig. 2.**6**).

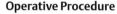 A prerequisite for this operation is the clear exposure of the septum in the middle of the operative field. It contains the cricopharyngeus muscle.

The diverticulum is cleaned of any food rests which might have collected. It is then inspected endoscopically and through the microscope. Moistened swabs are

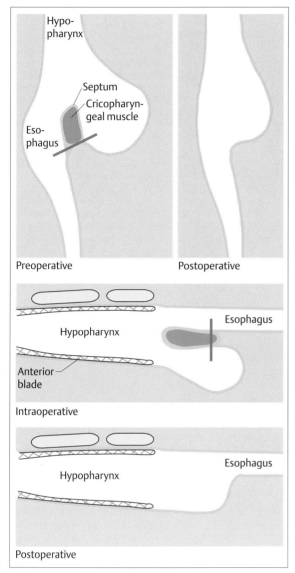

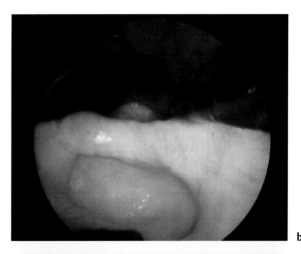

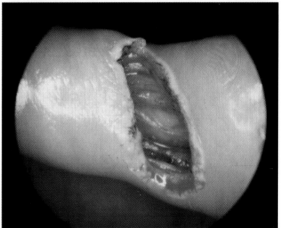

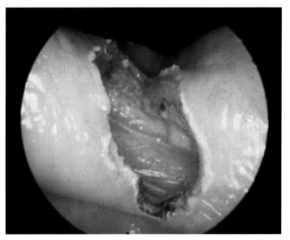

introduced to protect the esophageal mucosa from any accidental injury with the laser beam. The septum is then transected exactly in the midline with low power (approx. 5 W), and under high magnification of the microscope (Fig. 2.**6b–d**). During the careful dissection of layer after layer with the laser, the different tissue structures can be identified at the respective level of dissection and the mucosa and the transverse fibers of the cricopharyngeus muscle can be seen to separate and retract laterally. A V-shaped wound results. Bleeding is usually minimal and rarely is it necessary to use electrocautery for smaller vessels. The laser incision ends approximately 5 mm before the fundus of the diverticulum is reached. In very large diverticula a transection in several sessions can be contemplated (van Overbeek, 1994). Weerda (1988) recommends sealing of the raw mucosal edges along the esophagus and the remaining fundus with fibrin glue. We, however, do not use this technique.

Abb. 2.**6** Hypopharyngeal diverticulum. Diagram of preoperative, intraoperative, and postoperative anatomical relations. **a** During transection of the septum between esophagus and diverticulum, the fibers of the cricopharyngeal muscle are divided up to the indicated line. **b** The ridge formed by the cricopharyngeal muscle is demonstrated through the diverticulum scope. The diverticulum can be seen below; the anterior blade placed in the esophagus is shown above. **c** Transection of the mucosa and the musculature with the laser under microscopic control. **d** Situation at the end of the procedure. The bar of tissue has been almost completely removed.

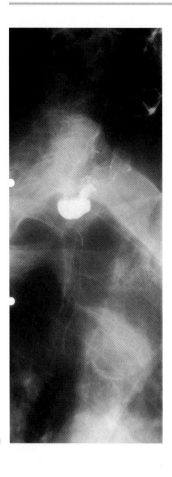

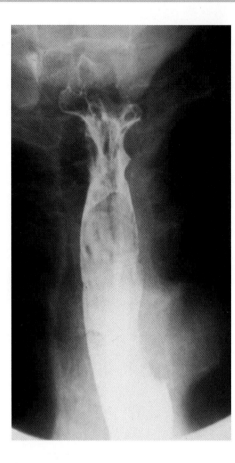

a

b

Fig. 2.**7**   Radiological imaging of hypopharyngeal diverticulum. **a** Preoperative Barium swallow, showing a Zenker's diverticulum at the typical site. **b** Postoperative control after 5 days. Dorsally a small pouch is still demonstrated with slightly delayed passage of contrast. There is, however, no residual pooling of contrast. **c** Two years after the operation, the Barium swallow shows a normal passage of contrast in this 86-year-old patient. No obstruction or delayed passage is noted in the proximal esophagus. The patient is symptom free. These radiographs were taken at an outlying hospital and kindly made available to us.

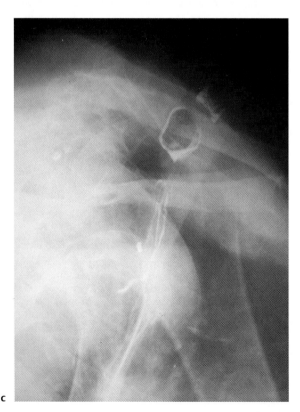

c

Postoperative Measures

Rudert, van Overbeek, and Weerda are very experienced surgeons in this field. Their recommendations (Rudert, 1995; van Overbeek, 1994; Weerda, 1988) regarding perioperative antibiotic prophylaxis, postoperative nasogastric feeding, and type and timing of postoperative radiologic investigations (Fig. 2.**7b** and **c**) differ considerably. Our policy, like that of the above-mentioned authors, is based on our own experience:
— Perioperative antibiotics or single preoperative dose;
— Rarely is there a need for a nasogastric tube;
— Patients are kept on intravenous fluids and nil per mouth for 24 hours, after which they receive a fluid diet for some days and then a soft diet for approximately another week;
— A chest radiograph is taken on day one postoperatively;
— A contrast swallow study is performed after 6 weeks.

Risks and Complications

Intraoperative: Hemorrhage and perforation. If the transection is carried out strictly in the midline, more severe bleeding can be prevented. We do not usually request any preoperative angiographic studies.

Postoperative: Secondary hemorrhage, surgical emphysema, mediastinitis (infection occurs as result of perforation). By applying the above-mentioned cautionary measures, the risk of postoperative complications is (very) low.

Advantages of the Endoscopic Laser Operation

The minimally invasive procedure is of shorter duration and has a lower morbidity for the patient. The complications associated with an open approach through the neck are avoided. These include, for example, infection, hematoma, recurrent nerve palsy, wound dehiscence, surgical scar.

Other advantages are a low complication rate, little pain, short hospital stay, no tendency to stenose, and a patient who is often completely free of symptoms. However, it must be mentioned that the recurrence rate is slightly higher in cases undergoing endoscopic surgery. The success is thus not as guaranteed, as it is with the transcervical approach. If, however, a discrete residual or recurrent diverticulum is demonstrated radiographically, a second procedure is not indicated in a patient with little or no symptoms

Laser Microsurgery for Benign Diseases of the Larynx

Indications:
- Congenital lesions:
  - laryngomalacia,
  - cyst, laryngocele, hemangioma,
  - stenosis.
- Acquired lesions:
  - nodule, polyp, cyst, (intubation) granuloma,
  - venectasia, varicosity,
  - (Reinke's) edema,
  - therapy-induced edema (postoperative conditions or after radiotherapy),
  - amyloidosis,
  - papilloma, hemangioma,
  - keratosis, leukoplakia, hyperplasia,
  - webs and stenosis,
  - bilateral recurrent nerve palsy.

The pseudotumors of the larynx are benign lesions and usually well circumscribed. Their development is often associated with an inflammatory process or a functional abnormality. They are most commonly found in adults but can also occur in children.

Diagnosis. Before any phonosurgical procedure, a thorough assessment should be made by a speech pathologist. A stroboscopic examination is important to evaluate the frequency and quality of the mucosal wave on the vibrating vocal fold. The findings on stroboscopy should be documented on video with a camera connected to the endoscope. A preoperative phonetogram is highly desirable (see Chapter 5, p. 124ff.).

Technical prerequisites. If the CO_2 laser is to be used in phonosurgery, certain technical prerequisites have to be met. Of particular importance is a good micromanipulator which can focus the laser beam to a focal spot size of 0.8 mm diameter. In general the use of a microspot micromanipulator (diameter of focus down to 0.3 mm) is not necessary. It will, however, improve the precision of certain procedures, for example, resection of vocal cord nodules. Unsatisfactory surgical results should not and cannot be blamed on the laser being an inappropriate tool for phonosurgical procedures. They are usually due to the lack of experience (unnecessary resection of healthy tissue is also possible in conventional microsurgery of the larynx) and inadequate technical equipment and instrumentation.

Vocal Cord Nodule

Vocal cord nodules are commonly the result of inappropriate use of the voice. Patients classically show the symptoms of functional dysphonia. Soft, sessile nodules are commonly distinguished from hard nodules. In children the nodules are often situated in the middle of the vocal fold, whereas in adults they are mostly located in the area between anterior and middle third of the cord. In the pediatric age group the soft nodules usually regress during puberty and in adults these soft lesions can usually successfully be treated by means of voice therapy. Soft nodules that are resistant to conservative therapy and hard fibrotic nodules should be treated surgically. The indication for surgery should be made by the speech pathologist.

Operative Procedure

The vocal cords are exposed through a closed, small-caliber laryngoscope. The use of the microspot micromanipulator and low power settings make the precise ablation of the lesion possible, with maximum preservation of healthy tissue as well as the vocal ligament at the base of the nodule. Fibrous nodules should be grasped with a cupped forceps during the resection and routinely submitted for histological examination. Early nodule formation and soft lesions can be treated with vaporization alone. For this purpose a moist gauze swab or a protector is placed under the vocal fold. The laser beam is directed so that it hits the nodule medial to the free margin of the vocal cord. With this technique, no damage can be inflicted on vocal cord mucosa or vocal ligament by the incident laser beam.

It is safer to aim the beam tangentially just medial to the nodule, i.e., the glottic aperture. This "shaving" technique considerably reduces the danger of injuring the vocal ligament.

Postoperative Treatment

Voice rest should be prescribed until the wound on the vocal fold has completely healed. The wound usually heals within approximately 2 weeks. Long-term results are largely dependent on the success of speech therapy in treating the underlying functional dysphonia.

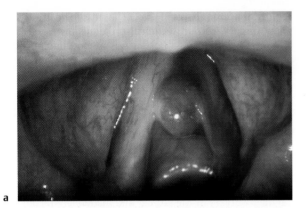

a

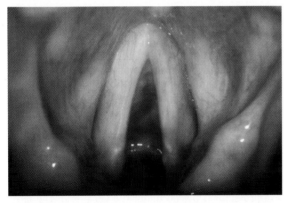

b

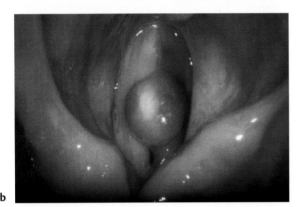

c

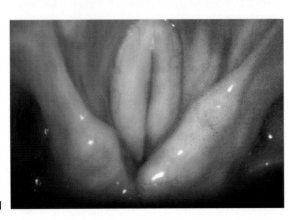

d

Fig. 2.**8**   Hemangiomatous polyp of the right vocal cord (endoscopic view, 90° telescope). Because of the simultaneous finding of a hematoma (the patient is on Warfarin therapy and has a history of voice abuse) conventional resection was not performed at another center. **a** Preoperative during quiet respiration. **b** Preoperative during phonation. **c** Postoperative during respiration. **d** Postoperative during phonation. After 3 weeks, the right vocal cord is well healed although still mildly erythematous. Complete glottic closure and normal vibration (stroboscopically proved) make normal phonation possible.

Polyps

Polyps are commonly unilateral and originate from the free edge of the vocal cord. Causative factors of significance are voice abuse and chronic inflammation. A vocal cord polyp will always require surgical removal, since spontaneous remissions are not to be expected. The polyp must always be submitted for histological examination and must not be vaporized. Rare benign tumors or an early glottic carcinoma are thereby excluded.

Operative Procedure

The vocal folds are exposed through a closed laryngoscope. To protect the distal mucosa, a moist gauze swab is introduced subglottically. The polyp is then grasped with a cupped forceps and retracted medially. This brings the cord mucosa under tension and the vocal ligament becomes visible. The mucosa is subsequently incised and the polyp completely resected. If a feeding vessel is noted in an angiomatous polyp under the microscope, it is primarily coagulated with the laser. At the end of the resection all that is left is a linear defect in the epithelium at the free edge of the vocal fold.

Postoperative Treatment

About 2 weeks postoperatively, the epithelial defect will have completely healed (Fig. 2.**8**) and the patient can again make normal use of his/her voice. If there is no underlying functional voice disorder, speech therapy is not necessary.

Laryngoceles and Cysts

Internal Laryngoceles

Internal laryngoceles are dilatations of the laryngeal ventricle, which is lined with respiratory epithelium. They may contain air or mucoid secretions and can extend into the false cord or even up into the aryepiglottic fold.

Operative Procedure

The supraglottis is exposed through a bivalved laryngoscope under general anesthesia. The mucosa overlying the laryngocele is incised in the area of the false cord or aryepiglottic fold, and the smooth outer surface of the lesion is defined. Finding the air- or mucus-filled bag is facilitated by the bloodless field left after the laser incision through the mucosa. The cele can then be opened and any secretions suctioned out. This will collapse the structure and complete excision down to its origin in the sinus of Morgagni is now possible. Extension of the internal laryngocele through the thyrohyoid membrane into the soft tissues of the neck results in a mixed laryngocele. In these cases the lining of the laryngocele can be followed into the soft tissues of the neck.

Cases of purely external laryngoceles should be managed via an external approach.

Cysts

Retention cysts are the most common lesions. They are caused by inflammatory processes resulting in an obstruction of the excretory duct of submucous glands. Their predilection sites are vocal cords, false cords, aryepiglottic folds and epiglottis. Complete resection is necessary to prevent a recurrence.

Operative Procedure

The cyst is visualized through a closed laryngoscope under general anesthesia. The mucosa overlying the cyst is incised and grasped with a fine forceps. The cyst is then peeled out in toto.

(Intubation) Granulomas

Intubation granulomas can be unilateral or bilateral. They are classically located on the vocal cord at the vocal process of the arytenoid cartilage. These lesions should not be resected before 4 weeks after the intubation, as spontaneous healing by separation from the underlying mucosa can occur. In rare instances an earlier ablation may be necessitated by symptoms of dyspnea or serious voice disturbances.

Operative Procedure

Another intubation should be avoided. Resection during a short apneic phase or with a jet ventilation technique is the preferred modality of treatment. The glottis is exposed through a closed laryngoscope, the granuloma grasped with a cupped forceps, and resected at its base. Unnecessarily wide exposure of the arytenoid cartilage, which is immediately under the mucosa, should be avoided. Recurrences can occur even after careful resection of a granuloma with the CO_2 laser. These are probably caused by persistent inflammation of the perichondrium in the area of the vocal process.

Ablation of *contact granulomas* is rarely indicated. Speech therapy and psychotherapy are the primary modalities of treatment according to the suspected causes of this condition. The surgical technique is the same as that for intubation granulomas.

Chronic Inflammation

Reinke's Edema

Reinke's edema is commonly a bilateral condition. Causative factors of importance are voice abuse and chronic inflammatory processes, mostly related to the inhalation of cigarette smoke.

Operative Procedure

The vocal folds are exposed through a closed laryngoscope. The laser is set at low power for the incision of the mucosa overlying the edema. Following this incision, the medial mucosal flap is held with a cupped forceps and the edema fluid with its mucoid substances is suctioned from Reinke's space. The excess mucosa is carefully resected with the CO_2 laser and the remaining mucosa is draped back. The mucosal cover of the free edge of the vocal cords is thus largely preserved. The advantage of the laser procedure lies in significantly reduced bleeding from the inflamed mucosa, when compared to conventional resection with microscissors. The mucosa over the edema may, however, contain vessels of more than 0.5 mm diameter which cannot be reliably coagulated with the laser beam. To achieve hemostasis in these cases, the application of a gauze patty soaked in an epinephrine solution might be necessary. Coagulation with monopolar electrocautery should be avoided.

Reinke's edema does not usually extend into the anterior commissure. Provided a good surgical technique is used, both vocal folds can thus be operated on in one session, without the danger of web formation.

Wound healing after excision is protracted due to the underlying chronic inflammation and takes 3–4 weeks. The removal of excess tissue results in incomplete glottic closure immediately after the excision with the consequence of temporary dysphonia. The patient must be counseled accordingly and should always undergo speech therapy after the wound has completely healed. The prognosis regarding voice improvement and recurrences is largely dependent on the patient's smoking habits and the intensity and level of competence of the administered speech therapy.

Chronic Hyperplastic Laryngitis

Smoking is often the underlying cause of chronic inflammation of the larynx. Other inhaled substances (e.g., dust, solvent vapors) or "endogenous" factors, such as chronic sinusitis or continuous mouth breathing, can also be of pathogenic importance. The characteristics of the *chronic-catarrhal variety* on macroscopic inspection are redness and mild thickening of the mucosa of the vocal folds and false cords. The initial treatment is conservative. Nevertheless, the condition can progress and change into a *chronic-hyperplastic laryngitis*. This form is characterized by edema, an increase in submucosal connective tissue, and hyperplastic epithelial lining with or without cellular dysplasia. The hyperplastic lesions can present on the vocal cords,

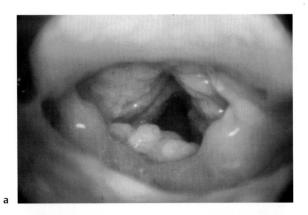

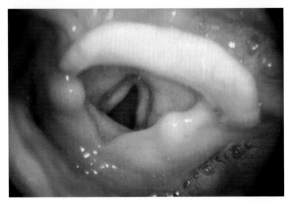

Fig. 2.**9**   Marked chronic hyperplastic laryngitis. **a** Preoperative findings. **b** Condition after extensive laser excision of all the hyperplastic changes. (Endoscopic view, 90° telescope).

Often an outflow of secretions from the submucosal glands can be observed during this mucosectomy. The glands are partially removed with this peel, resulting in a reduction of the mucoid secretions once complete healing has taken place. In the next step the mucosa of the vocal cords is peeled off. Care is thereby taken to preserve the vocal ligament and the mucosa of the anterior commissure. A strip of intact mucosa should also be left behind in the laryngeal ventricle to prevent adhesions between true and false cords.

Postoperative Treatment

Primary extubation is possible even after extensive resections of almost the entire mucosa of the endolarynx (for which we use the term "endolaryngeal mucosectomy"). Inhalations are given postoperatively. After 4–5 weeks, complete reepithelialization of the larynx can be expected (Fig. 2.**9**). The voice is usually markedly improved following this surgery. Further improvement can be achieved by speech therapy. The long-term prognosis is dependent on the successful avoidance of the causes.

Papillomas

Papillomas can occur at any age. Most commonly they become manifest in childhood between the ages of 1–3 years. Children under the age of 1 year presenting with papillomas have, however, been reported. The diagnosis is made with the flexible endoscope or at microlaryngoscopy. Small and uncooperative children with chronic and particularly progressive dysphonia must be examined under general anesthetic.

The recurrent disease is caused by the human papilloma virus (HPV6, HPV11). Causal treatment does not exist and repeated microsurgical ablations, aimed at maintaining an airway and improving the quality of the voice, are the mainstay of therapy. The growth rate of the papillomas, and hence the frequency of necessary interventions, vary greatly from patient to patient. The majority of laryngologists today consider the precise, bloodless, and tissue-friendly resection using CO_2 laser the treatment of choice. Based on early experience with the CO_2 laser in the 1970s, new hopes were raised that the recurrence rate could be brought down to lower levels. However, after more than 20 years of experience with this method, it has been realized that these expectations could not be fulfilled. We have been using the laser technique since 1979. Before this, conventional removal with cupped forceps, microscissors, and suction diathermy was performed (1973–1978). A retrospective analysis of the course of the disease in our patients showed prolonged intervals between operations in the group treated with the CO_2 laser. However, higher rates of disease-free patients could not be achieved by the method. The prolonged interval between ablations is thought to be the result of the more precise and more complete removal with the CO_2 laser (Fig. 2.**10**).

the false cords, and the epiglottis in various degrees of severity. All degrees of cellular dysplasia can thereby occur simultaneously within the epithelium. Chronic hyperplastic laryngitis can give rise to the development of a carcinoma due to the effect of field cancerization. For diagnostic purposes punch biopsies from different areas are often recommended in these cases, yet a "false negative" biopsy can still miss severe dysplasia, carcinoma in situ, or even a microinvasive carcinoma. We prefer the complete excision of the macroscopically diseased mucosa. This makes a safe diagnosis possible and promotes healing of even the more severe cases of hyperplastic laryngitis through regeneration of the mucosa (Fig. 2.**9**).

Operative Procedure

General anesthesia and endotracheal intubation are used for this operation. In severe cases of diffuse hyperplastic laryngitis, the larynx is exposed through a bivalved laryngoscope for resections in the supraglottis and through a closed laryngoscope for the procedure on the vocal folds. In the first step the hyperplastic mucosa in the supraglottic area is peeled off. A precisely focused beam with medium power is used.

Operative Procedure

In any patient with papillomas the examination must not only focus on the larynx, but a full panendoscopy should also be performed to exclude extralaryngeal manifestations of papillomatosis in trachea, bronchi, pharynx, and esophagus. At the beginning of the procedure, the areas of papillomatosis are localized using rigid telescopes with angled optics. Special care should be taken in the assessment of laryngeal ventricles and subglottis. We prefer endotracheal intubation for this procedure also in small children. This is the safest possible form of airway control and ventilation and allows the surgeon to perform an undisturbed operation. We use a semi-tubular laryngoscope in children and a bivalved laryngoscope in adults. In cases of extensive disease the larynx is visualized through the laryngoscope and the resection is started on the epiglottis and the false cords. A closed laryngoscope is later introduced to remove the papillomas from the vocal cords and the subglottis. Papillomas on the medial aspects of the arytenoid cartilages, in the interarytenoid area, and caudal to this are best reached after temporary removal of the endotracheal tube. The resection is then performed in the apneic phase. Access can also be gained by using the closed laryngoscope to displace the endotracheal tube toward the anterior glottis. The temporary use of jet ventilation also allows the resection of papillomas in this region. We used this latter technique extensively during the 1970s.

! The resection proceeds from cranial to caudal to prevent areas of papillomatosis being missed during the procedure. Small lesions might become squashed by the laryngoscope, making them flat and invisible at a later stage during surgery. In addition, small hemorrhages from a proximal focus of papilloma could affect the visibility and lead to incomplete resection of the more distal lesions.

The laser beam may be slightly defocused. Low power settings should be used and the resection limited to the mucosa affected by papillomas. Small islands of normal mucosa should be preserved between the papilloma lesions to promote quicker reepithelialization of the endolarynx. However, the papillomas should be ablated as completely as possible to achieve prolonged symptom-free intervals.

⚡ Great care should be taken in cases of bilateral disease of the vocal cords with involvement of the anterior commissure. Especially in children, the resection in this area should be conservative. Small foci of papillomas should rather be left behind to prevent adhesions in the anterior commissure. Fibrinous membranes can be removed by gently swabbing the anterior commissure and the formation of a web thus prevented. In children, however, this would have to be done under general anesthesia.

In patients with frequent recurrences in the anterior commissure and subglottis, we only opt for complete resection of papillomas and scar tissue if webs have

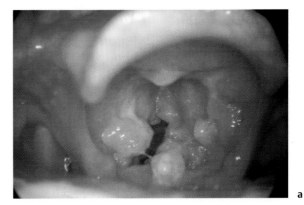

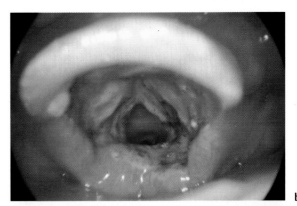

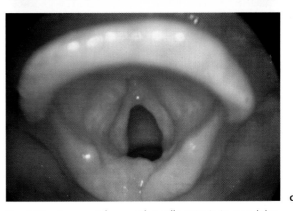

Fig. 2.**10** Recurrent laryngeal papillomatosis in an adolescent before and after microscopic laser resection (endoscopic view, 90° telescope). **a** Extensive recurrence of papillomas in the endolarynx. **b** Fibrinous membranes on the extensive wound surface after laser treatment. **c** The larynx is completely healed 4 weeks after the resection with the laser.

already developed. In adult patients, regular swabbing of the anterior commissure under topical anesthetic is performed approximately twice weekly as prophylaxis against scar formation (Fig. 2.**11**). In children, the follow-up treatment also consists of swabbing of the anterior glottis. This is performed under short general anesthesia with ketamine but without endotracheal intubation.

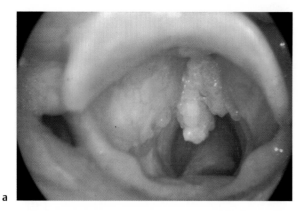

a

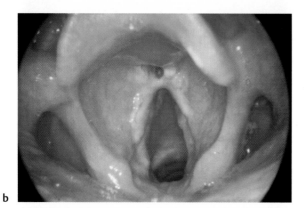

b

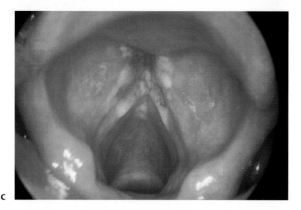

c

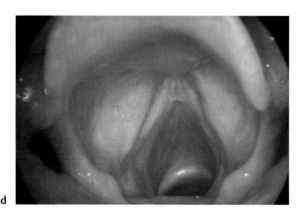

d

Fig. 2.**11** Recurrence of laryngeal papillomas in the anterior glottis and subglottis (endoscopic view, 90° telescope). **a** Preoperative microlaryngoscopic findings. **b** A few days after the laser resection the possibility of a web formation must be entertained. The fibrin layers on the wound are seen to cross the anterior glottis and the subglottis. **c** The formation of a synechia is prevented by active swabbing of the anterior larynx and removing the fibrinous material. Residual fibrin is noted anteriorly in the supraglottic and glottic area on both sides. **d** Healed endolarynx without signs of recurrence of papillomas. Anteriorly a small web of scar tissue is noticeable.

During resection of the papillomas with the CO_2 laser, the incision itself hardly ever causes any bleeding. More commonly, small hemorrhages result from the squeezing of papillomas between the cups of a forceps. Monopolar electrocautery is better avoided, since deeper-lying tissue structures might be damaged in the process. Usually the application of cotton wool balls soaked in an epinephrine solution is sufficient to achieve hemostasis. If coagulation is deemed necessary, bipolar electrocautery should be used.

A good surgical technique is of particular importance for this operation. It will help to preserve the tissue layers under the mucosa and thus prevent unnecessary scar formation.

Primary extubation after the operation is possible even in cases of extensive resections. This may be assisted by the administration of a single dose of a corticosteroid (e.g., 3 mg/kg prednisolone). Perioperative antibiotics are not indicated. Even wider resections can be performed as outpatient cases or during short hospitalization.

> In our opinion a tracheotomy should be avoided under all circumstances.

In over 25 years we have only had to perform a tracheotomy once. This was in a 2-year-old child who had to undergo surgery every 3–4 weeks for severe recurrent papillomatosis. After the tracheotomy the child developed massive recurrent disease in the trachea. Despite repeated therapy with different interferons, the disease could only be brought under control at the age of 12 years after more than 50 laser applications.

Hemangiomas

Among the laryngeal hemangiomas one distinguishes between the predominantly capillary hemangioma of early childhood and the cavernous variety in the adult patient.

Capillary Hemangiomas in Infants

This hemangioma typically presents as a well-circumscribed, reddish swelling in the posterior subglottis, most commonly on the subglottic belly of the vocal cord (Fig. 2.**12**). Hemangiomas that originate in the posterior commissure and extend along the subglottic bellies of both vocal cords are more rarely encountered as are lesions extending into the anterior commissure.

Operative Procedure

At the beginning of the operation the trachea and the main bronchi are inspected with a 0° or 25° telescope to exclude other hemangiomas. After endotracheal intubation, the larynx is exposed through a semi-tubular laryngoscope. The hemangioma is ablated step by step using a precisely focused beam and low power. The capillary vessels of the lesion are thereby coagulated without any spillage of blood. The endotracheal tube is removed temporarily if it obstructs the view, and the operation continued during an apneic phase. As an alternative, jet ventilation can be employed. A unilateral hemangioma can be entirely ablated in this fashion and the vocal fold almost fully preserved at the same time (Fig. 2.**12**). In order to prevent stenoses from scar formation, large bilateral hemangiomas require a modification of this approach. Initially only a unilateral ablation should be performed to create an airway of adequate lumen. The second side can then be addressed during a second operation.

Postoperative Treatment

In very small children prolonged intubation for 1–2 days and the administration of corticosteroids and antibiotics have proved to be successful. After extubation, the breathing of humidified air can help to reduce the formation of fibrinous membranes, which may cause symptoms of respiratory distress. If stridor occurs despite local and systemic treatment, a second microlaryngoscopy should be performed. The fibrinous membranes and granulation tissue, which might have formed, are then carefully removed with the laser.

The Nd:YAG laser, if used in a noncontact fashion, has the advantage that no open wound results. The hemangioma "shrinks," but the depth of penetration of the laser beam is difficult to estimate.

Cavernous Hemangioma in Adults

The hemangiomas of adulthood are mostly cavernous. They can be removed with the CO_2 laser if they are pedunculated or limited to circumscribed areas of the supraglottis. The feeding vessels, which can be quite large, must be dissected out during the operation. They are coagulated or ligated with vascular clips. The vascular tumor can then be gradually dissected from the surrounding tissue. Postoperatively the patient should remain intubated until the following day. Close monitoring of the patient is necessary during the first postoperative days, because of the possibility of a secondary hemorrhage. The additional use of the Nd:YAG laser can be helpful in the management of the rare, extensive vascular malformations which stretch to involve large parts of the larynx as well as oropharynx and hypopharynx.

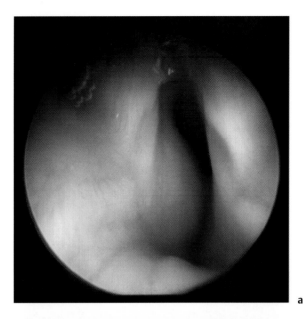

a

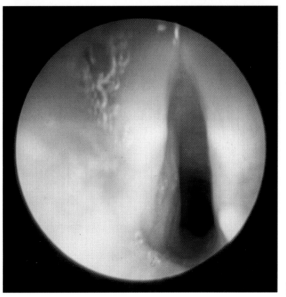

b

Fig. 2.**12** Subglottis hemangioma in a newborn. **a** Preoperative laryngotracheoscopy under general anesthetic. **b** A few weeks after partial resection with the CO_2 laser. The airway was satisfactory.

Endolaryngeal Glottic Enlargement in Bilateral Recurrent Nerve Palsy

The purpose of the operative enlargement of the glottis is to find a balance between airway patency and voice quality. On the one hand, an airway must be created to provide unobstructed breathing even during physical activity and to allow the closure of a tracheostoma, if this has become necessary. On the other hand, the impairment of voice quality should be kept to an absolute minimum. It must be noted, however, that none of the numerous modifications of external or endolaryngeal operations achieves a compromise that is satisfactory for both airway and voice.

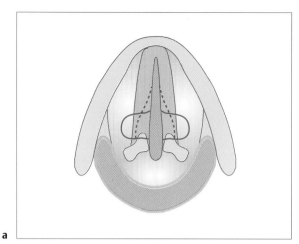

a

Fig. 2.**13**   CO$_2$-laser bilateral posterior cordectomy in bilateral recurrent nerve palsy. **a** Schematic drawing of the procedure. An adequate lumen is usually achieved by bilateral resection of the posterior third of the vocal cord including the vocal process. The body of the arytenoid cartilage is preserved in this operation. The resection must reach far enough laterally (red line) and inferiorly to achieve a satisfactory result for airway and voice quality. The formation of granulation and scar tissue is unpredictable and varies from patient to patient. Usually we can expect a result as shown on the dotted line and on the endoscopic view during respiration (**c**).
Endoscopic view (90° telescope) of the larynx after laser treatment during phonation (**b**) and during respiration (**c**). Breathing could be improved maintaining the voice quality because of preservation of the vibrating parts of the vocal folds.

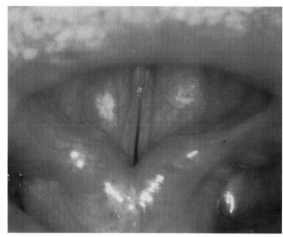
b

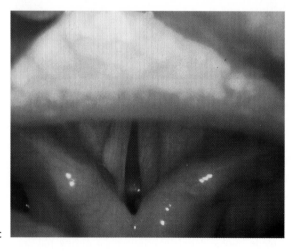
c

Diagnosis

The diagnosis should be confirmed by an electromyographic study of the involved laryngeal muscles, preferably the vocalis muscle. Stroboscopic examination with video documentation and a voice analysis are desirable as preoperative investigations. A lung function test (body box plethysmography) performed before the operation and again postoperatively allows objective assessment and documentation of the success of the treatment. The procedure should be performed at the earliest 6 months after an operation on the thyroid which caused the bilateral palsy of the vocal cords.

Operative Procedure

The unilateral microsurgical laser arytenoidectomy is the most commonly performed endoscopic procedure. Numerous variations of endoscopic laser surgical management exist. Simultaneous removal of the vocal fold, total cordectomy and posterior cordotomy are all modifications of this procedure. We see a number of advantages in the bilateral resection of the posterior part of the vocal cord in the area of the vocal process (posterior cordectomy). This is the surgical technique of choice, advocated by Burian and Höfler (1979) and, if individually modified, is the closest one can get to a compromise between an adequate airway and a good functional voice. In this operation the glottis is only widened posteriorly. Since large parts of the arytenoid cartilage are preserved, no postoperative problems with aspiration occur, as they do after complete endoscopic arytenoidectomy. The morbidity of the operation is low. A tracheotomy is not necessary if the patient has not already had one preoperatively. We have been using this technique since the beginning of the 1980s.

The posterior glottis is exposed through a closed laryngoscope under general anesthesia. In the first step the vocal ligament and the musculature anterior to the vocal process are transected (Fig. 2.**13**). In the second step a transection of the ligamentous and muscular structures immediately anterior to the body of the arytenoid cartilage is performed. The soft tissue lateral to the vocal process is subsequently resected. The preservation of the vibrating part of the vocal cords is of utmost importance for postoperative voice quality.

Perioperative Measures

The patient is given a single dose of prednisolone and is extubated immediately. Perioperative antibiotics are not routinely administered. Wound healing is generally complete after 4 weeks.

Postoperative Treatment

After surgery, the extensive formation of fibrin on the wound can lead in some patients to respiratory distress. In these cases we try to remove the membranes by gently wiping the wound with a cotton wool applicator under topical anesthesia. If excessive formation of granulation tissue occurs, this may necessitate a second procedure. The patients must be counseled accordingly before the operation. If the achieved widening of the glottis is not adequate after wound healing has been completed, the operation can be repeated. A more liberal resection of the vocal cords can be considered.

It is difficult to predict the individual reaction of a wound regarding the formation of granulation tissue and scarring. In some cases a second operation becomes inevitable, despite initial "over-correction," to finally achieve a satisfactory glottic opening. Since an endoscopic operation with the laser is less strain on the patient than the extralaryngeal techniques, and in most cases primarily succeeds, we consider it the procedure of choice for bilateral vocal cord palsy.

Stenoses of the Larynx

Types:
– Congenital membranous stenosis (webs) of the anterior commissure,
– Glottic or subglottic, partial or circumferential stenoses after intubation,
– Treatment-induced supraglottic or glottic stenoses (e.g., after partial resection and/or radiotherapy for larynx carcinoma),
– stenoses of various causes (idiopathic, following acid or alkali ingestion, burns, specific diseases, rare proliferative diseases, and others).

Supraglottic stenoses, for example after conventional supraglottic partial laryngectomy, usually have a good prognosis. Nevertheless, wide excision of the scar tissue is necessary. Several operations are commonly required to achieve the desired result. The resection starts immediately inferior to the tongue base. Tissue is generously resected with the laser anteriorly and laterally, and an "over-correction" is aimed for (Fig. 2.**14**). Posteriorly the resection extends to just anterior to the arytenoid cartilages. The preservation of the function of the arytenoids is of particular importance for normal postoperative swallowing. Extensive combined supraglottic and glottic stenoses with impaired movement of the arytenoid cartilages are usually the result of surgery or radiotherapy. A complete rehabilitation of respiratory and swallowing function is difficult (repeated endoscopic laser procedures with insertion of stents) or impossible to achieve.

Primary and secondary *webs of the anterior glottis* are very successfully treated with the CO_2 laser (Fig. 2.**15** and 2.**16**). The block of scar tissue is excised in toto with low power and preservation of the vocal ligament. To prevent the adhesions from reforming, a resection of the anterior commissure is made in the shape of a keyhole onto the inner surface of the thyroid cartilage. In the past we vigorously swabbed the anterior glottis through this gap under topical anesthetic two to three times per week following the surgery. A special solution of cortisone, an antibiotic, and alpha-chymotryptase can be used to soak the cotton wool used for the swabbing. Wiping the fibrinous exudate prevents the cords

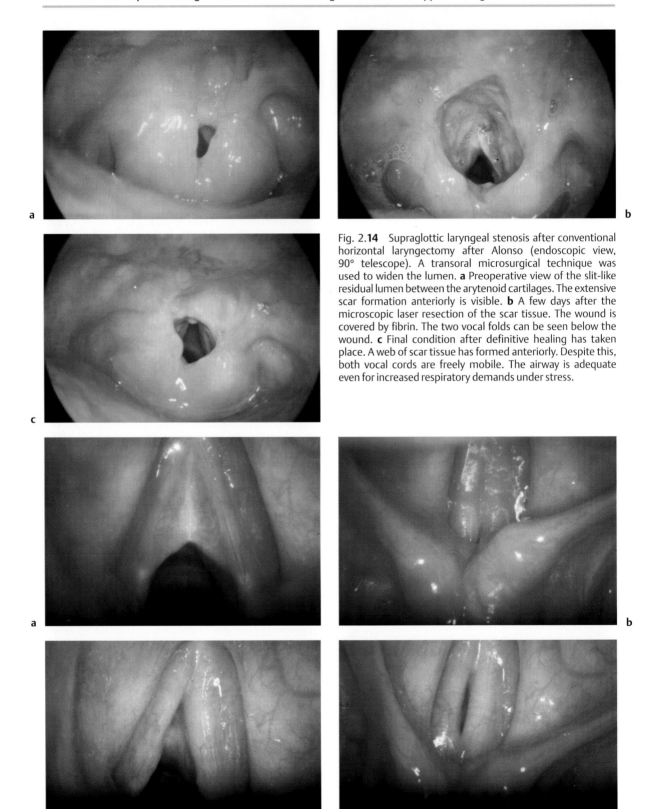

Fig. 2.**14** Supraglottic laryngeal stenosis after conventional horizontal laryngectomy after Alonso (endoscopic view, 90° telescope). A transoral microsurgical technique was used to widen the lumen. **a** Preoperative view of the slit-like residual lumen between the arytenoid cartilages. The extensive scar formation anteriorly is visible. **b** A few days after the microscopic laser resection of the scar tissue. The wound is covered by fibrin. The two vocal folds can be seen below the wound. **c** Final condition after definitive healing has taken place. A web of scar tissue has formed anteriorly. Despite this, both vocal cords are freely mobile. The airway is adequate even for increased respiratory demands under stress.

Fig. 2.**15**   Endoscopic photos (90° telescope) of a congenital anterior glottic web (**a** and **b**). Findings after single laser treatment and successful swabbing to prevent the formation of adhesions (**c** and **d**). Postoperatively stroboscopy shows that the full vibratory function of both vocal cords has been maintained. Residual hypofunctional symptoms are amenable to speech therapy.

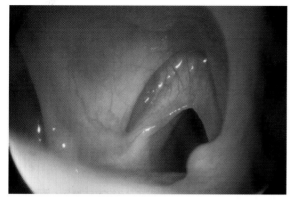

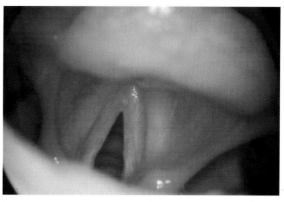

Fig. 2.**16** Postoperative web before and after microsurgical laser transection. **a** Preoperative findings of a membranous web of the anterior and partially the middle glottis.

b Eight weeks after laser excision of the web through the 90° telescope.

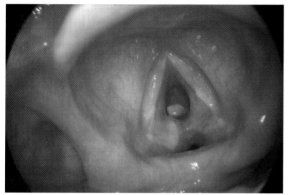

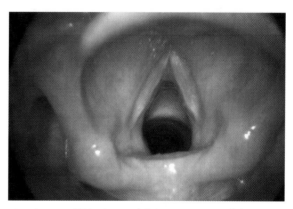

Fig. 2.**17** Posterior glottic stenosis following intubation. **a** Marked adhesions from granulation tissue in the posterior glottis between the vocal processes after long-term intubation. A small residual lumen can still be seen posteriorly

at endoscopy (90° telescope). **b** Laser resection of the granulation and scar tissue results in an almost normal larynx.

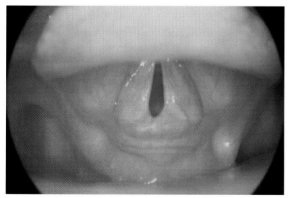

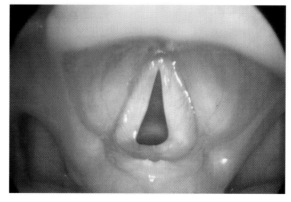

Fig. 2.**18** Interarytenoid fibrosis (posterior web) after short intubation (40 minutes). **a** Preoperative finding (endoscopic view, 90° telescope). The residual lumen of the glottis is restricted to 2–3 mm due to posterior adhesion. **b** Situation after single laser transection and excision of the scar in the posterior glottis. The lumen has been enlarged to 3–4 mm.

The elderly patient was satisfied with the resulting airway. She no longer experienced stridor at rest. In order to achieve a more pronounced enlargement in the posterior region, a stent or a cartilage graft would have to be inserted after laser surgical excision of the scar. However, the patient refused this procedure.

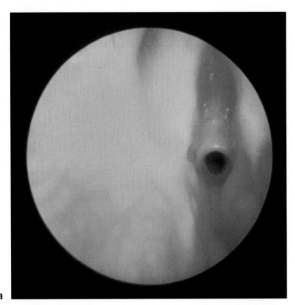

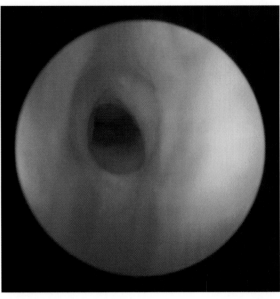

a

b

Fig. 2.**19**   Subglottic stenosis in an infant. a Preoperatively a circumferential subglottic stenosis can be seen. It was the result of long term-intubation. b Four weeks after laser excision of the anterior membrane of scar tissue, an adequate lumen at the level of the cricoid cartilage was achieved to allow decanulation of the patient.

from sticking together, and the repeated interruption of wound healing leads to delay in epithelialization. If there is excessive formation of granulation tissue, a laser-surgical ablation might be indicated. Children can also be treated with this technique. The postoperative swabbing of the anterior commissure must then be done under a short general anesthetic, usually without endotracheal intubation. An alternative to the regular swabbing is the use of a silastic sheet secured with a penetrating suture (Friedrich, 1996). This technique may be combined with an autogenous free oral mucosal graft. We have recently obtained good results with this technique.

Posterior glottic stenoses have a good prognosis if there is only a bridge formation between the vocal processes (interarytenoid adhesion of Benjamin) (Fig. 2.**17**). The situation is less favorable in cases of interarytenoid fibrosis. Splitting of the fibrotic band with the laser or extensive resection of scar tissue in the posterior glottis without stenting are often only partially successful (Fig. 2.**18**).

In the *subglottis* endoscopic laser treatment only has a chance of success in the rare membranous, sickle-shaped stenosis following intubation. Usually several endoscopic laser procedures are necessary to achieve the desired result (Fig. 2.**19**). In the case of an extensive, circumferential or lengthy scar stenosis a therapeutic attempt with the CO_2 laser is indicated to alleviate the airway obstruction and prevent a primary tracheotomy. Long-term success, however, is only possible if a stent is inserted, and even then remains doubtful. Endoscopic treatment is contraindicated if a collapsed cricoid cartilage is part of the pathology. These stenoses must be managed with a conventional laryngotracheoplasty technique using cartilage or bone grafts and an external approach.

3 Endoscopic Microsurgical Laser Treatment of Malignant Diseases of the Upper Aerodigestive Tract

Preoperative Diagnosis

This chapter covers those aspects of diagnosis that are common to all the malignancies in the various regions of the upper aerodigestive tract. Table 3.1 gives a survey of the diagnostic methods and procedures used for staging of carcinomas in the oral cavity, pharynx, and larynx.

The minimum requirements for preoperative staging are endoscopy, ultrasound (US) examination of the neck, PA and lateral chest radiographs and, in advanced tumors, upper abdominal US. The results of these investigations will help to make decisions about the initial treatment.

Initial Investigation of Suspicious Lesions in the Upper Aerodigestive Tract

When a suspicious mucosal lesion has been detected, the following procedures are carried out to decide on the diagnosis (benign, premalignant, or malignant)
- Inspection of oral cavity and oropharynx using the operating microscope;
- Endoscopy of larynx and pharynx with a 90° telescope with magnification;
- Video and/or photo documentation (reprints for patient's record and oncology file);

- Smear cytology;
- Biopsy for histology
  - prior to radiotherapy and/or chemotherapy,
  - prior to extensive partial resections or radical resections,
  - if cytology is negative!

In cases of atypical necrotic slough or ulceration, granulomatous diseases such as tuberculosis, fungal infections, and syphilis as well as the possibility of HIV/AIDS must be considered in the differential diagnosis. This is especially so if
- there is no history of smoking or alcohol abuse,
- in high-risk groups, or
- when additional symptoms of a systemic or specific disease are found.

Swabs for microbiological examination are taken to rule out the above-mentioned diseases. Stains for fungi and fungal cultures must be specifically requested. Serological tests and a chest radiograph are part of the routine investigation in these cases.

The nature and extent of further pretherapeutic investigations are determined by:
- The mode of therapy (organ preserving surgery, radiotherapy and/or chemotherapy),
- Intention of treatment (whether curative or palliative).

Table 3.1 Investigations for the diagnosis and staging of tumors of the upper aerodigestive tract

Aims	Investigations
Primary tumor (T) – Type of lesion (differential diagnosis) – Tumor extent • Superficial • Deep	Endoscopy, smear for cytology, histology (biopsy, excision biopsy) Endoscopy, optional: imaging modalities Contrast-Spiral CT, MRI (e.g., in cases of infiltration of the soft tissues of the neck or the large vessels)
Cervical metastasis (N) – N0?, N+? – degree of metastatic disease	Routine US (B-scan) CT and MRT in special circumstances (e.g., skull base infiltration). If a CT or MRI examination of the primary tumor is performed, the neck is obviously evaluated at the same time.
Distant metastasis, (M)	Chest radiograph, US examination of the upper abdomen In case of suspicion: CT mediastinum and thorax MRI of abdomen (liver) In certain cases: imaging by scintigraphy
Second primary	Panendoscopy

Staging of Locoregional Disease

If an early lesion is present or suspected, we do *not* consider computed tomography (CT) or magnetic resonance imaging (MRI) indicated before the diagnostic/therapeutic laser excision has been performed.

Even in more extensive lesions, routine preoperative imaging is not performed for the following reasons:

- Our approach is primarily one of endoscopic resection initially;
- At the time of endoscopy the tumor extension is determined under direct microscopic vision while the lesion is resected, organ preservation being the major objective.

For assessment of nodal spread, we prefer US to CT or MRI as an initial examination.

The value of imaging for the preoperative assessment of larger tumors is in determining local spread into the neck. (Fig. 3.**1**). For instance, spread to the carotid sheath would preclude the transoral approach. Although such disease could be removed by a combined open and transoral technique, this has, in our experience, had such a poor prognosis that such patients are better managed by radiochemotherapy.

The value of imaging is greatest for staging before radiotherapy or for making a decision whether to perform radical or organ-sparing surgery. Generally, imaging improves the assessment of tumor extension, helps to identify neck metastases, and gives more information on the extent of cervical metastases. One must, however, be aware of the limits of imaging in this staging process. The comparison of imaging findings with objective results from histological examination of surgical specimens highlights the *shortcomings* of these diagnostic tools (Fig. 3.**2**).

Overestimation of the size of the tumor is possible if the tumor is surrounded by inflammatory changes, edema, or fibrosis (false positive). Submucosal tumor spread or cartilage invasion, on the other hand, can result in an underestimation of the extent of the lesion (false negative).

The resulting effects on management decisions can be demonstrated by two extreme situations in the larynx. Problems with movement artifacts occur regularly during imaging of the larynx and make the interpretation more difficult. Presumed infiltration of cricoid and/or thyroid cartilage on CT or MRI (false positive finding) in

Table 3.**2**   Comparison of CT and MRI for diagnosis of oncological disease in the upper aerodigestive tract

Relevant structure	Evaluation (with regards to special aspects)
Oral cavity and oropharynx	*MRI is superior to CT* due to better soft tissue contrasts and less artifacts from dental fillings
Tongue, especially base of tongue	Actual submucosal extent of tumor?
Lateral wall of oropharynx and hypopharynx	Parapharyngeal extension?
Tonsillar fossa	Infiltration of soft tissues of the neck?
Inferior hypopharynx, postcricoid, and esophageal inlet	Infiltration of paraesophageal tissues?
Larynx and hypopharynx	*CT is better*
Medial wall and apex of pyriform sinus, postcricoid area	Destruction of cricoid cartilage?
Posterior wall of pharynx	Infiltration of vertebral bodies?
Oral cavity	Destruction of the mandible?
Carcinoma of the anterior commissure with subglottic extension	*CT equal to MRI* Infiltration or destruction of thyroid/cricoid cartilage? Extralaryngeal growth with break-through – via cricothyroid membrane – via thyroid cartilage
Cervical lymph drainage	*CT usually superior,* N-staging is, however, possible with MRI. The choice depends on the imaging method chosen for the primary tumor. Detection of clinically occult metastases (N0 becomes pN+)
In advanced cervical metastatic disease	Skull base involvement, encroachment of carotid artery, infiltration of carotid artery?

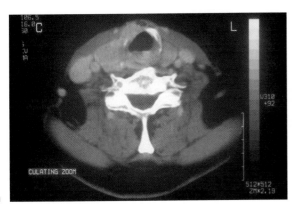 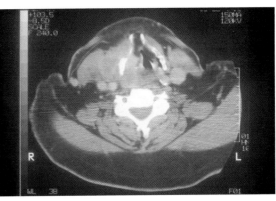

a   b

Fig. 3.**1** Contrasted CT scans of the neck showing some contraindications for transoral microsurgical laser resection of tumors in larynx and hypopharynx. **a** Extensive larynx carcinoma with spread across the midline. The entire posterior and right lateral wall is infiltrated by tumor (main origin). The tumor has broken through into the soft tissues of the neck all the way into the subcutaneous fat. There is suspicion of destruction of the cricoid cartilage by tumor and infiltration of the right thyroid lobe. **b** Large right-sided hypopharynx tumor involving the larynx and breaking through into the soft tissues of the neck. There is extension into the prevertebral space and infiltration of the right ala of the thyroid cartilage up to the midline.

a carcinoma of the anterior glottis with subglottic extension may suggest that a laryngectomy is required (*"overtreatment"*). Missed invasion of a cartilage could lead to *"undertreatment"* in the form of radiation alone. Pretherapeutic understaging of a tumor, erroneous interpretation of test results, or failure to perform preoperative imaging may result in unpleasant intraoperative surprises.

Should the surgeon be faced with an unexpectedly large tumor during an attempted partial resection, the option of radical surgery immediately or at a later stage still exists. Postoperative radiotherapy or combined radiation and chemotherapy are yet another possibility aimed at organ preservation.

Pretherapeutic overestimation of tumor extent results in an unnecessarily radical operation with the sacrifice of an organ (e.g., laryngectomy, layngopharyngectomy). Conversely, the omission of a curative operation in favor of primary radiotherapy and/or chemotherapy may result in a worse prognosis. Fortunately, these diagnostic dilemmas are relatively rare.

☞ The transoral microsurgical technique using the laser makes an operation possible, which addresses the primary tumor. It aims at the preservation of the organ and thereby preserves its function. This can be achieved without extensive preoperative imaging, which even in the very best hands is not completely reliable.

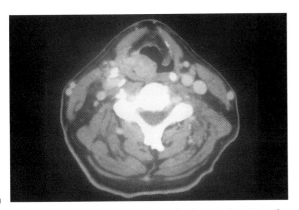 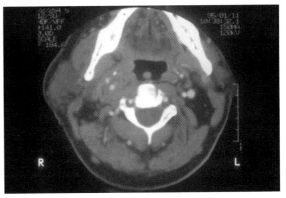

a   b

Fig. 3.**2** Examples of false positive findings at imaging. The limitations of the imaging modalities (in this case CT) are demonstrated. Wrong interpretations during tumor staging are possible, which can result in wrong therapeutic steps being taken. **a** Large polypoid tumor of the right aryepiglottic fold with involvement of the medial wall of the pyriform sinus. The impression is created that the hypopharyngeal lesion has infiltrated the soft tissues of the neck. Here the CT does not allow an exact delineation of the tumor from healthy tissue. **b** Tonsil carcinoma with advanced cervical metastases. The impression is created of a tonsil carcinoma that has infiltrated into the neck in the sense of a continuous lesion. This would require a combined approach from inside and outside. However, during the diagnostic laser tonsillectomy it was shown that the primary tumor had not infiltrated the neck tissues.

Panendoscopy

Aims

Endoscopy of the upper digestive and respiratory tract aims at
– defining the extent of the primary tumor, and
– detecting a second primary lesion.

Indications, Timing, and Technique (Flexible and/or Rigid)

Indications

- Proven carcinoma of the upper aerodigestive tract, for which curative surgery is planned.
- Further investigation of organ-specific symptoms and findings:
  - symptoms such as cough, sputum production, hemoptysis, dysphagia,
  - suspicious chest radiograph.
- Patients with premalignant conditions of the oral cavity or larynx. In these patients, risk factors such as smoking habits, alcohol consumption, occupation, and age must be considered.

Timing of Panendoscopy

a) Simultaneously with the diagnostic pretherapeutic staging; in the case of advanced tumors when the indications for curative laser surgery are still uncertain.
- A biopsy of the primary tumor is taken when:
  - smear cytology is negative, or
  - radiochemotherapy and/ or radical surgery are planned,
- during assessment of the extent of the primary tumor.

b) At the beginning of the curative laser resection.

- When no positive histology or cytology has been obtained, frozen-section histology is performed.

Operative Procedures

1. Laryngotracheobronchoscopy and subsequent endotracheal intubation
2. Inspection through the microscope of oral cavity and oropharynx
3. Microlaryngoscopy and hypopharyngoscopy
4. Esophagoscopy

After ventilating the patient with a mask we usually expose the larynx with the McIntosh or a semi-tubular laryngoscope during short muscle relaxation. Larynx, trachea, and bronchi are examined endoscopically with a 25° or 30° telescope. In our experience this examination provides adequate access to all bronchial segments (including the bifurcations of the upper lobes) which are sites of predilection for synchronous or metachronous bronchial carcinomas.

Alternatively, we use a rigid ventilating bronchoscope and inspect the bronchial tree with 0° and 90° optics or via the endotracheal tube with a flexible bronchoscope. Bronchoscopy with ultrathin flexible endoscopes for the exclusion of tumors in more distal bronchi, which is of importance to the pulmonologist in investigating specific symptoms, is not required for routine elective endoscopy.

The difficult intubation. Anatomical considerations can present obstacles for rigid bronchoscopy. In bulky, obstructive laryngeal tumors, tissue trauma and bleeding should be avoided. For this purpose the relaxed patient is ventilated through a mask. The procedure is essentially as above, except that the larynx is not visualized with rigid endoscopes. In these rare cases, the *flexible endoscope* with an endotracheal tube passed over it can be used for intubation. Subsequently, the flexible bronchoscope is used to examine the distal trachea, and larger bronchi are then inspected. If indicated, a bronchial lavage can be performed at the same time. If there is massive obstruction of the larynx, a jet ventilation probe can be passed into the trachea under visual control. Alternatively, a jet cannula is inserted through the cricothyroid membrane for temporary ventilation, while the tumor is being debulked with the laser.

The endoscopy of the respiratory tract is followed by a *microscopic inspection* of the oral cavity (aided by gags and tongue depressors) and the immediately accessible areas of the oropharynx (tonsil and palate). For the microscopic examination of the *oropharynx* (tongue base and vallecula), *hypopharynx*, and *larynx* we commonly use the distended laryngopharyngoscope. It provides better exposure of the base of tongue and the vallecula, including the supraglottis, and enables the surgeon to expand the pyriform sinus and the postcricoid area. This is a prerequisite for a thorough examination of the hypopharynx and the esophageal inlet. Finally, an *esophagoscopy* is performed. Usually we employ a rigid endoscopic technique; a 0° telescope is carefully introduced and air is insufflated to expand the esophagus. If rigid endoscopy of the esophagus is difficult for anatomical reasons, we perform a flexible esophagoscopy.

A general rule for elective diagnostic procedures is not to force any endoscope, rigid or flexible. According to the principle "primum non nocere," the procedure should be aborted if problems arise in order to prevent, for example, a perforation of the esophagus. The risks must obviously be weighed up for every individual patient.

Suspicion of a Second Primary in the Upper Aerodigestive Tract, Bronchi or Esophagus and the Consequences for the Curative Resection of the Primary Tumor

Second primary in the upper aerodigestive tract. The lesion, if resectable, is removed microsurgically like the primary tumor. If the lesion is only discovered under general anesthetic, it will usually be an early-stage tumor.

Second primary in the esophagus or bronchi. In these cases it is of significance if the second cancer is an early-stage tumor or an advanced lesion. The prognosis of the second tumor and the T-stage of the primary are important factors for making the decision to proceed with the laser resection of the first tumor. A second primary tumor in bronchi or esophagus may have a bad prognosis. Generally, it is our practice that the primary tumor should be resected regardless of the second tumor when the resection can be performed without excessive risk or without severe functional sequelae (e.g., aspiration). The aim here is to improve or at least preserve the patient's quality of life. This is particularly so if swallowing or airway can be improved.

> In principle, conventional radical procedures, such as laryngectomy, are generally not indicated in patients with a prognostically poor second primary in either the esophagus or bronchi.

The Concept of Function-Preserving Therapy for Carcinomas of the Upper Aerodigestive Tract

The surgical, oncological, and functional principles are the same for minimally invasive surgery as for more conventional resections. The primary concern is the complete resection of the tumor while every effort is made to preserve as much function as possible. At initial surgery the cancer is resected radically according to oncological principles and histologically clear margins are aimed for. At the same time the largest possible amount of healthy tissue that is not involved by tumor should be spared. This will preserve the anatomical integrity of the organ as far as possible and thereby provide the basis for the greatest possible preservation of function.

> The principle is to minimize the surgical morbidity while not compromising time-honored oncological principles.

Procedure

During transoral laser microsurgery, decisions are made in accordance with the local spread of the tumor. The tumor extension is clearly distinguishable under the microscope, and the lesion is resected until healthy tissue is found and an appropriate safety margin can be maintained.

Small and well-circumscribed tumors are excised en bloc. In larger tumors the cancer is transected to enable the surgeon to estimate the depth of tumor penetration. This can be seen on the cut surface under high magnification, and enables the surgeon to determine a clear surgical margin. Normally, sections through the tumor are made by the pathologist while examining specimens in the laboratory. The *intraoperative distinction between tumor and healthy tissue* can generally be made quite easily in untreated patients and particularly so in carcinomas of the larynx and hypopharynx. In cases of doubt histological confirmation from a frozen section can be obtained. If surrounding tissues are involved, such as cartilage or bone, they are included in the resection.

The aim of complete resection is achieved by variations in technique concerning the cutting instrument used and the surgical technique. In general a transoral approach is chosen primarily and the CO_2 laser is used as a cutting instrument under microscopic control.

Limitations of Transoral Laser Surgery

When examining the limitations of transoral microsurgery, mention is usually made of difficult exposure. Occasionally it may not be possible to expose the whole operative area with one single position of the laryngoscope, even when an adequately large laryngoscope is used. This is usually due to patient-related problems, but also depends on the experience of the surgeon. If adequate exposure is provided, there are, in principle, no *technical limitations* for transoral surgery. Any tumor is resectable by an appropriately experienced surgeon. The real technical limits of surgery are reached in cases of massive tumor infiltration into the soft tissues of the neck, where the access routes become a problem (Fig. 3.**1**). Should the surgeon encounter this situation, an external approach through the neck must be chosen to complete the resection. Closure of the resulting defect can be achieved by mobilizing parts of the neck musculature. If the tumor does not reach the proximity of the carotid sheath, a complete resection can still be performed from the inside. Conventional instruments should then be used for the dissection along large vessels. These can be clipped by the use of ligaclips with a special applicator (Fig. 1.**5d**). The wound should then be covered with collagen mesh and fibrin glue to protect the great vessels in the neck. A neck dissection should not be performed earlier than 8 days after this procedure. In our experience this has afforded sufficient protection to the great vessels in these cases, and no patients have suffered serious consequences.

The limitation of the endoscopic technique is not related to the oncological or technical aspects of obtaining clear margins, once sufficient experience has been achieved, but is rather reached by the severe *swallowing problems* that can occur postoperatively.

This problem may occur when both arytenoid cartilages or the esophageal inlet have to be sacrificed due to tumor infiltration. Such cases are fortunately relatively rare in our experience.

> ⚡ The main complication in far-advanced tumors that require an extensive resection is postoperative aspiration, which may be temporary or permanent.

The generally accepted oncological indications for conventional partial resections of larynx and hypopharynx, as well as for the organ-sparing transoral microsurgical techniques, are discussed in the sections on the respective organs. At this point it should be mentioned that some principles of cancer surgery which have been practiced for decades may no longer be valid today. This would include the paradigms that in extensive neck disease a partial resection of the organ bearing the primary tumor is not justified; and that in advanced primary tumors a radical neck dissection is always indicated regardless of the stage of nodal disease. It does not appear logical to radically remove an organ in patients who have advanced neck disease and therefore have a poor prognosis.

Securing Tumor Resection with Clear Margins

Any tumor surgery must subscribe to the principle of complete resection with clear surgical margins which can be documented histologically. This chapter addresses the problem of achieving and histologically documenting clear margins, which is of importance in local control. This involves the cooperation of surgeon and pathologist.

Recognition of Tumor Extent (Superficial and Deep)

The *microscopic view* and the cutting characteristics of the laser are properties which can be used to determine the extent of the tumor. The microscopic advantage, with its inevitably narrow margins, must be contrasted with the conventional approach, which attempts to achieve clear margins by sacrificing a large amount of normal tissue. Presently, however, it is still unusual for head and neck surgeons to employ the operating microscope for resecting tumors.

At high magnification *early carcinomatous changes and premalignant lesions* (severe dysplasia, carcinoma in situ, and microinvasive carcinoma) can be detected in the mucosa immediately adjacent to the carcinoma; this has been termed "field cancerization." The limitations of the operating microscope are obvious when compared to the histological assessment by the pathologist under much higher magnification. Mucosa that appears healthy under the surgeon's microscope might already harbor epithelial atypia. Another shortcoming of the operating microscope lies in the recognition of submucosal extension of carcinoma, which will be discussed at a later stage.

High magnification and low power (3–5 W) with a modern, high-precision CO_2 laser makes an almost char-free incision into normal tissue, especially when an acuspot or microspot control is used. The relatively *bloodless cutting* of tissues further improves the view and thereby the interpretation of the nature of the tissue. An experienced surgeon can differentiate benign from malignant with surprising precision. The *degree of carbonization* of the tissue occurring during the cut with the laser serves to identify tumor tissue. This applies equally to superficial tumors in the mucosa and to deep extensions of tumor such as submucosal spread or infiltration into surrounding musculature or to submucosal extension. These features enable the surgeon to extend the resection as required.

Surgical experience and the feedback from histological reports help to build up reasonable clinical accuracy in deciding to resect specific areas. If, for instance, a carcinoma of the vocal fold is excised with a safety margin of 2 mm within healthy looking mucosa and atypical carbonization of the tissue is noted or delayed separation of the tissues occurs, then the excision of a further 2 mm of mucosa is advocated. This tissue should be sent separately for histological examination. Practice has shown that the surgeon's suspicion is often confirmed by the pathologist's examination. It is generally acknowledged that this risk is even higher in carcinomas of the oral cavity and the oropharynx, where resection margins should be more generous. This is also the case with conventional "macroscopic" surgical techniques.

Increased tissue density or increased vascularization can render the assessment of the tissue reaction to the laser more difficult. Differentiating tumor from normal tissue can be difficult when glandular tissue is cut, for example, in the area of the false cord, the arytenoid cartilage, or the tongue base. Difficulties can also arise in highly vascular areas (inflammatory changes) and in scar tissue from a previous biopsy, operation, or irradiation. More pronounced carbonization during laser resection is also characteristic of these areas. Surgical technique, whether conventional or microscopic, is dependent on an appreciation of tumor extent, which in turn depends upon experience and additional information from imaging.

The "safety margin" using conventional surgical technique is essentially derived from excising well within healthy tissue (Fig. 3.**3b**). Structures surrounding the tumor, such as cartilage, bone, muscle, etc., are sacrificed to ensure this safety. While "overtreatment" is often unavoidable with this approach, "undertreatment" is still possible despite a generous excision. This would explain positive margins or local recurrences reported after conventional radical resections such as laryngopharyngectomy. The occurrence of a new cancer in the resected area as a cause of "local recurrence" must be considered a rarer situation.

Choosing and Keeping an Adequate Resection Margin

Macroscopic resection margin ("safety margin") refers to the distance between the line of resection and the macroscopically visible tumor on the mucosal surface. A number of factors are of importance in deciding where and how the incision should be made. This includes organ-specific factors (vocal cord vs. hypopharynx vs. tongue), but also smoking and drinking habits and the effect of surgery on function.

After many years of smoking and alcohol abuse there is an increased risk of dysplastic or malignant changes in the mucosa surrounding the tumor and indeed for the entire mucosal surface of the upper aerodigestive tract through the field cancerization effect. Second primary tumors can be synchronous or metachronous. The risk of submucosal finger-like extensions of a tumor is greater in the tongue than in the vocal cord. In the hypopharynx the resection of an extra 5–10 mm of mucosa will not influence function, whereas the taking of an additional 1–2 mm of the vocal fold will have a decisive influence especially on a professional voice user. It is also of significance whether the tumor is superficially spreading or deeply infiltrating. Finally, clinical experience will determine the difference in approach to, for example, leukoplakia and an ulcerating tumor, allowing a greater safety margin for the latter.

The same principles regarding safety margins, which are used in traditional tumor resections can be applied to laser surgery. The recommendations range from 5 mm to a few centimeters, depending on tumor site and author. We are of the opinion that, due to the prognostic implications of a positive margin, surgical overtreatment is often performed. The rate of local recurrence is related to the rate of regional recurrences which will increase the rate of tumor-related mortality.

The actual extent of the tumor is unknown especially in larger tumors and can only be estimated. Hence, the conventional surgeon will choose as wide a safety margin as possible to resect the tumor with clear margins. Uninvolved structures such as musculature, cartilage, and bone are sacrificed with potential functional implications. The laser-surgical resection of larger tumors implies cutting through tumor to visualize the deep borders of the cancer. This enables the surgeon to individually adjust the safety margin so that the tumor is resected with a clear margin and function is preserved at the same time.

We choose a resection margin of *1–3 mm for the area of the vocal cord*, bearing in mind the possibility of premalignant and microinvasive disease not macroscopically evident. The reasons for this decision are discussed in Chapter 3, p. 47. For all other areas, such as *supraglottis, oral cavity, oropharynx, and hypopharynx*, we prefer a margin of at least *5 mm* for small superficial tumors and 5–10 mm for larger tumors and those with a deeply-infiltrating growth pattern. The reason for this is the greater risk of early changes in the vicinity of the

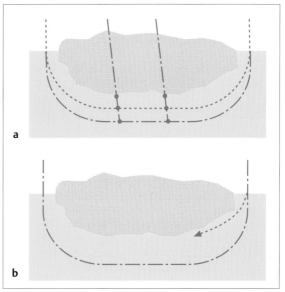

Fig. 3.**3**   Lines of resection for laser microsurgery and conventional surgery for squamous cell carcinoma of the upper aerodigestive tract. **a** During laser surgery, cuts are made through the tumor. In the previously untreated patient, the differentiation between tumor and "not tumor" is usually easily possible. The borders of the tumor can be recognized by the surgeon and the individual distance from the lesion is then chosen. The cut surface of the tumor is inspected intraoperatively. In conventional surgery only the pathologist gets to see this. It enables the surgeon to better assess the submucosal extensions of the tumor and its topographical relation to neighboring structures. **b** The resection line during conventional surgery shows the wide excision of a tumor. The surgeon does not know the actual distance between the resection line and the tumor border. The lesion is excised with an intended wide margin of healthy tissue around it. The second line closer to the tumor is a reminder of the danger of getting too close to the tumor. This is a distinct possibility after the mucosa has been incised and a tangential cutting technique is used for the deeper dissection.

tumor, which are difficult or impossible to detect clinically and the greater propensity of these tumors for submucosal spread.

Special situations. In some areas we consider a more liberal resection necessary. These include floor of mouth, tongue, and palate, since they harbor a greater potential for carcinomatous changes in the immediate vicinity and submucosal spread of tumor. For this and other technical reasons, at least a complete tonsillectomy is performed for tonsillar carcinomas regardless of the size of the primary tumor.

In the upper digestive tract the resection of a few more millimeters of mucosa has no significant negative effects on healing and function. This makes a more generous excision of the tumor and the keeping of a wider safety margin possible. The special circumstances surrounding the resection of extensive tumors in the proximity of cartilage, bone, or large cervical blood vessels will be discussed in more detail in the sections dealing with the treatment of tumors in the individual areas.

So far the choice of the adequate resection margin was discussed with special regard to criteria that are specific for organ and tumor. However, a correct *cutting technique* with the laser is another prerequisite for maintaining an adequate safety margin. The type of laser and the technique of cutting also play a major role in achieving tumor resection with histologically proved clear margins.

The use of a first-generation laser can result in a broad line of carbonization, which can result in diagnostic problems in the interpretation of the adequacy of the resection margin. It is therefore better to use a newer-generation laser with a narrow band of vaporization, since the factor of importance in the histological assessment is the width of normal tissue between the tumor and the laser resection line. This means that a safe distance must be kept from the tumor independent of the cutting characteristics of the laser to obtain the histological confirmation of clear margins.

The more modern CO_2 lasers, especially with acuspot or microspot, leave a very thin line of carbonization of 25–50 micrometer (Fig. 3.**11**). The advantage is less impairment of the histological examination. The negligible width of the cut is another contributing factor to the maximum preservation of tissue and function. This has greater relevance in areas such as the vocal cord, where a few millimeters of additionally resected tissue have a significant effect on function.

The surgeon's cutting technique with the laser is another important factor. A clean cut, making use of a narrowly focused laser beam contrasts with several parallel cuts resulting in a wide incision. The individual need for safety on behalf of the surgeon plays a role as well. Intersurgeon variability will result in different margins being taken.

Proof of clear margins in all three dimensions is necessary for the complete resection of a tumor. Compromise of the resection margins may occur by cutting tangentially with the laser in the deeper-lying areas of the resection. The same applies to conventional surgical techniques. Kleinsasser and Glanz (1984) pointed out that a faulty cutting technique enhances the risk of resecting too closely to the tumor (Fig. 3.**3b**). This risk is, for instance, relatively low for superficially growing, well-defined glottic carcinomas. Carcinomas of the tongue, on the other hand, usually tend to have an infiltrating growth pattern and submucosal extensions. If tissue is encountered that raises the suspicion of tumor, the resection must be extended by a few millimeters. In cases of doubt about the margin of the resection, an excisional biopsy is necessary from the edge of the wound for frozen-section or definitive histological examination.

Technique of Resection and Histological Processing

Small tumors (vocal cord up to 5 mm, oral cavity up to 10 mm) can be excised en bloc (Fig. 3.**4**, 3.**5a** and 3.**7**). The margin for the resection is chosen individually and must take patient factors and tumor site (vocal fold vs. tongue) into consideration. The histological processing follows tumor and site-specific criteria.

Care must be taken intraoperatively not to compromise the distance between tumor and resection line by cutting tangentially during the deep dissection.

☞ A small excision specimen allows for histological examination of all resection margins (Fig. 3.**10**). The procedure for specimens from the vocal cord is described in detail in Chapter 3, p. 49ff.

Tumors of the oral cavity and the oropharynx with a maximum diameter of 10 mm are also resected in one piece, although with a wider safety margin of 5–10 mm. This also applies to tumors of the supraglottis and the hypopharynx, where small lesions are even less common.

The resection of smaller carcinomas of the oral cavity, oropharynx, and hypopharynx basically follows the method described by Mohs for skin tumors and modified by Davidson et al. (1988) for mucosal tumors of the upper aerodigestive tract. All surfaces parallel to the excision line are examined histologically by this method. The Mohs surgeon uses a scalpel and the operating microscope to cut thin slices from all the lateral resection margins of the specimen not only from the mucosal edges. The surface facing away from the tumor is stained with a blue marking pen (Fig. 3.**4**). The thin tissue slices from the margins are fixed in formalin and embedded in paraffin in such a way that sections can be made perpendicular to all surfaces facing away from the tumor and subsequently examined histologically. The surgeon also marks the deep resection margin on the remaining main tumor specimen. The central parts of the tumor are sectioned in slices of approximately 3 mm by the pathologist. They are embedded and cut perpendicular to the mucosal surface so that depth of infiltration and deep resection margins, as well as differentiation of the tumor can be assessed.

Extra biopsies taken with a biopsy forceps from the wound surface have been advocated. They are either examined as a frozen section or by definitive histology but have not proved successful. The uncertainties of this method are not due to the technique of frozen section. According to the literature a discrepancy between results from frozen section and paraffin embedded cuts only occurs in about 2% of cases (Gandour-Edwards et al. 1993). The uncertainty of the method lies, however, in the arbitrariness of the biopsies. They are not representative and have little diagnostic value. Hence, it is not recommended to base the assessment of the margins (positive or negative) on punch biopsies taken from the wound surface. For this purpose the edges of the specimen embedded in paraffin should be exam-

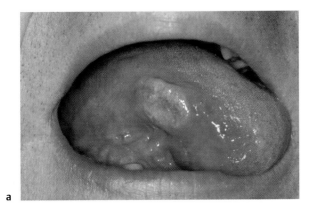

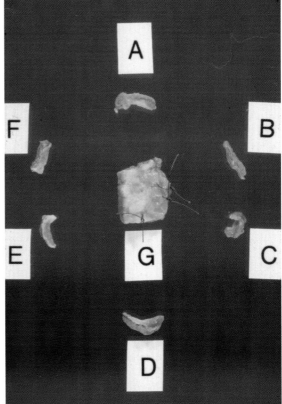

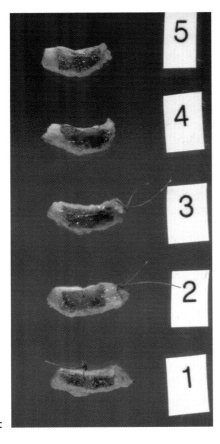

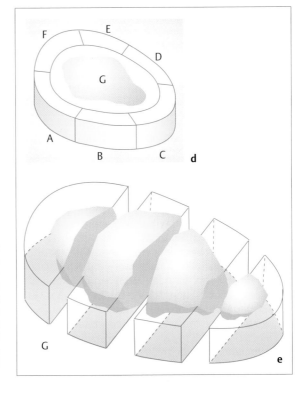

Fig. 3.**4** **a** Circumscribed carcinoma of the lateral tongue on the right. The tumor is excised with a margin of 5–10 mm. **b** and **d** Under the microscope, the surgeon obtains representative, three-dimensional specimens from the resected block of tissue (**b**, A–F). The surface facing away from the tumor is marked blue. These specimens from the margins should be free of tumor. The main specimen (G), which contains the tumor in the middle, is serially sectioned by the pathologist (**c** and **e**). The basal resection margin, which is stained blue, must be free of tumor. The grade of differentiation and the depth of infiltration is determined on the main specimen.

ined or alternatively further representative excsions obtained from the wound surface in the place of the punch biopsies.

Depending on the size of the tumor (vocal fold 5 mm, other sites more than 10 mm) and its location, we cut one or more sections through the tumor. In a larger T1a tumor of the vocal cord (Fig. 3.**15**) one vertical section is usually sufficient. In a tumor of the tongue base, with a diameter of 15 mm, we make two cuts through the lesion that are perpendicular to one another and cross in the middle.

Arguments Against an En Bloc Resection of Larger Tumors

In the beginning of our transoral microsurgical experience, we attempted to resect even more extensive tumors in one piece using the laser. We could demonstrate that endoscopic partial resections of larynx and hypopharynx are indeed technically possible with an en bloc technique. We have, however, also encountered a number of disadvantages of this method and therefore modified our surgical technique accordingly in the early 1980s and decided on the unconventional method of "block-wise" resection of tumors.

Impaired view during dissection. Parts of the tumor that have already been mobilized can reach the size of the diameter of a small laryngoscope. Despite retraction and often relatively free mobility of these tissue segments, this may lead to an incomplete resection, with tumor tissue being left behind or to the unnecessary resection of healthy tissue.

No knowledge of the actual safety margin. In the attempt to resect the tumor in one piece the surgeon cannot accurately judge the extent of tumor infiltration in the depth of the wound. This is analogous to conventional resection techniques. Although the dissection takes place under the microscope in tissue that is seemingly healthy, i.e., free of tumor, the surgeon is unable to identify whether the resection line is too close to the tumor, at an adequate distance from the tumor, or too far into healthy tissue (Fig. 3.**3b**).

For these reasons we introduced the unconventional surgical procedure of cutting through the tumor. This has become our method of choice for these more extensive cases. Understandably, this goes against the generally accepted principles of surgical practice in head and neck oncology. Initially there was a great deal of resistance to this even within our own department, however the refusal of many patients to agree to a radical operation became a challenge. With these organ-sparing principles in mind we could ethically and morally justify this unusual and previously untested surgical technique. There is no technical alternative to the resection of very extensive tumors via the endoscope. The tumor must be resected in several pieces similar to the debulking of large cancers during palliative, symptomatic laser treatment (Fig. 3.**5c**). The real justification for this policy was obtained retrospectively by the successful results that were achieved.

There are no indications that there is an increase in late regional or distant metastases due to laser incisions through tumor. This may be explained by the sealing effect of the lymph vessels which has been observed (Werner, 1993)

Tumor patients have been treated by this technique of resection developed by us from the early 1980s onward. The long-term follow-up of these patients has confirmed our belief in this unconventional laser surgical procedure. The rate of regional recurrences and distant metastases for comparable tumor stages is not higher for laser resections than after conventional resections. Finally, the tumor-related and overall survival rates correspond to those after conventional surgery and are in some cases even better.

Dissecting Technique and Histopathological Processing

Under high magnification the surgeon recognizes the tumor extension into deeper tissues by cutting through the tumor. He can then individually adjust the borders of the resection (Fig. 3.**16**). If the line of resection gets too close to the tumor, it can immediately be made wider. If suspicious areas are encountered, additional tissue can be resected and the excised material sent for an immediate examination by frozen section. Alternatively, the results of definitive histology can be awaited and further tissue resected in a second operation. After another vertical incision through the tumor, the deep resection can be performed under direct vision; the piece of tissue containing the tumor can then be removed (Fig. 3.**5**).

The surgeon subsequently marks the deep resection margin on the specimen. A marking pen is used under microscopic vision and great care should be taken with this task. It facilitates the orientation of the pathologist, who is then able to give a reliable answer to the question of adequacy of the resection margins. This marking is even more important when pieces of tissue are submitted that are taken from the depths of the wound and thus lack an epithelial surface which might help with the orientation of the pathologist (Fig. 3.**5c**).

The surgeon must keep a record in the form of a diagram of the precise origin of all individual specimens resected and submitted to the pathologist. A good topographical orientation postoperatively allows a detailed comparison of intraoperative and histological findings to be made.

The specimens are embedded and sectioned perpendicular to the surface of resection. Depth of infiltration, resection margins, and differentiation of the tumor are looked for. In certain cases the lateral (superficial) margins are marked. Usually, however, if there is doubt about the adequacy of the lateral margin, it is much safer to immediately resect a further 1–2 mm. The pathologist then examines these tissue sections as being either free of tumor, containing single nests of tumor cells, or being infiltrated by tumor.

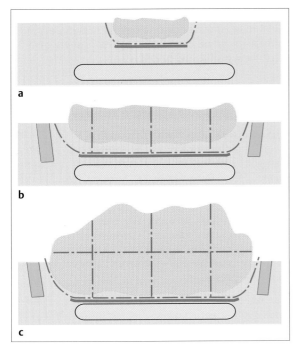

Fig. 3.**5** Examples of the resection technique. **a** A small, well-circumscribed tumor is excised en bloc. The histological work-up is done by serial sectioning. **b** A larger tumor is resected in several pieces. The basal margin is marked blue for better orientation of the pathologist. Additional specimens can be obtained by the surgeon from the anterior, posterior, and inferior resection margins to ensure the complete resection with margins of normal tissue. **c** In cases of exophytic and/or deeply infiltrating tumors debulking is initially performed in several pieces. The subsequent procedure is the same as described in b. The basal margins are marked blue. The yellow lines depict the site for facultative further specimens from the lateral margins.

Particulars of the Resection of Larger Tumors

Debulking of the tumor requires more power. Care must be taken not to cut too deeply into normal tissue with this powerful laser beam without adequate control and without good vision. The deeper the resection proceeds, the more difficult the orientation becomes. Surrounding structures such as large vessels, healthy tissue, but also the tumor margins are put at risk.

Clearly identifiable *tumor rests should always be left behind* during the debulking procedure. These remnants are easily distinguished at a later stage, when the final detailed resection with histological control is performed. Furthermore, the operation should be performed *with overlapping resection lines*, i.e., when a tumor remnant is removed, the cut is commenced in an area of the wound that has already been cleared of tumor in order to ensure complete resection.

Sometimes an area of the wound that has already been completely resected is found to look suspicious under the microscope after a prolonged operating time. The reason could be pressure from the laryngoscope or other influences, such as superficial hemorrhages. In this case a further slice of tissue should then be obtained from the area in question for histology.

The largest representative block of tissue is sent for histological examination. The resection margins being marked with a blue pen on their deep surface (Fig. 3.**5**), exactly as it has been described for medium-sized tumors (Chapter 3, p. 63ff).

The difficulties inherent in examining conventional specimens effectively apply to these specimens as well. Multiple step–sections need to be made and the adequacy of the pathological report is only as good as the effort expended and the experience of the pathologist.

Features of interest:
- Histological extent of tumor in three dimensions
- Depth of infiltration
- Adequacy of safety margin along all resection lines

These features are also of importance in the work-up of specimens of conventional surgical specimens. This is extremely labor-intensive for the laboratory. Specimens of larynx are possible exceptions to this rule (Kleinsasser 1987; Glanz 1984; Michaels and Gregor, 1982).

The orientation by the surgeon of the resection specimens is of crucial importance for the pathologist to be able to make a representative assessment. The tissue sections should be numbered, orientated with a blue marker on the resection margins and fixed, or sent for frozen sections in some cases. The effectiveness of the pathology report also depends upon the surgeon's liaison with the pathologist. Any additional information that the pathologist can get on the individual case is of great value. It must, however, be understood that the main responsibility lies with the surgeon, as it does with any conventional surgical technique. Pathologists can only comment on what is presented to them.

Postoperative Assessment

Basic requirements for this are:
- Operation notes
- Documentation of findings
- Intraoperative sketches
- Video documentation
- Interaction with the pathologist
- In cases of uncertainty, personal examination of specimens

The surgeon is faced with the following decisions:
- Immediate further resection
- Reassessment including laser biopsies after several weeks or
- Regular follow-up examinations

If a clearly positive margin is found by the pathologist, we try to perform a *wider resection* within a few days. This often happens at the time of the staged neck dissection. Any further resection is generally unproblematic and can be performed at any time, since the wounds are left open after laser resections and are not concealed by flaps. The wound is covered by fibrinous material at that stage. At the site of the positive margin an appropriately large piece of tissue is resected and the deep margin again marked. It can be difficult for the surgeon to differentiate between granulation tissue and residual tumor, especially when a strong inflammatory response is encountered. Immunohistochemistry to cytokeratin can be used for the histological evaluation and will make it possible to definitely distinguish between inflammatory and tumor cells.

When it is reported that the tumor comes close to the excision line, a number of factors must be considered in deciding on further resection. The following are of importance:
- Localization of the tumor (e.g., vocal fold versus tonsil)
- Size of the tumor (e.g., T1 versus T4)
- Intraoperative situation (e.g., clinically complete resection performed)
- Is further resection still possible, for example, in the area of the thyroid cartilage, or would the thyroid cartilage also have to be resected?
- Is there a high risk associated with further surgery, for example, resection in the proximity of the carotid artery?
- Would further operative intervention imply the loss of the last functional arytenoid cartilage?

These and a number of other factors must be critically weighed, when deciding on. When residual tumor may be present, the options are: immediate further surgery or a "wait and see" policy. In the latter case or after very large resections where the interpretation of the adequacy was difficult, microlaryngoscopic assessment with further laser resections, often combined with an elective neck dissection, should be made after 4–6 weeks. This endoscopic check-up serves to detect new malignant growths in the mucosa surrounding the original tumor, but is mainly performed to detect residual tumor. For this purpose it is frequently necessary to excise granulations or scar tissue that has already formed. This applies in particular to the regions where the initial resection was performed with a very narrow margin. Exact area and extent of the resection during this essentially diagnostic procedure depend on the local findings and also on the experience of the surgeon.

Postoperative Care

The examinations at follow-up should ideally be performed by the surgeons themselves. If this is not possible, an experienced colleague, who is also a oncological surgeon, should examine the patient. The frequency and the extent of the follow-up (endoscopy, video documentation, smears for cytology, ultrasound examination of the neck, etc.) are discussed in more detail in Chapter 3, p. 50ff. and p. 114f.

Advantages of Transoral Laser Microsurgery over Standard Therapy

The transoral approach. This approach obviates the need for a dissection through healthy tissue to gain access to the tumor, and also contributes to very limited blood loss. By preserving functionally important structures, such as cartilage, muscle, nerves, etc., a more rapid and effective rehabilitation of the patient is achieved. This is especially true with respect to swallowing after transoral partial resection of the supraglottic larynx, hypopharynx, and base of tongue using the laser, since both superior laryngeal nerves are generally preserved.

The use of the microscope. This enables the surgeon to expose the superficial and deep extension of the tumor more precisely. In addition, the microscopic view facilitates the detection of any further dysplastic or neoplastic changes of the mucosa surrounding the visible tumor (field cancerization).

The specific cutting properties of the CO_2 laser. The high-precision CO_2 laser makes an almost char-free incision into normal, nontreated tissue. The relatively bloodless cutting of tissue occurring during the incision with the laser serves to identify tumor tissue. The relatively bloodless cutting of tissues not only provides a better view of the surgical field and excellent conditions for the intraoperative assessment of the tissues with enhancement of surgical accuracy, but also decreases blood loss. The hemostatic effect of the CO_2 laser during transection of tissue can be combined with immediate conventional monopolar or bipolar electrocautery of larger vessels. The patient does not require any blood transfusion, not even for extensive resections.

"Blockwise resection." The unconventional surgical technique of cutting through larger tumors during the resection and removing the tumor blockwise has a distinct advantage. It allows the surgeon to inspect the cut surface of the tissue, which is usually only the privilege of the pathologist during sectioning of the specimen. There are no indications that there is an increase in late regional or distant metastases due to laser incisions through tumor. This may be explained by the sealing effect of the lymph vessels which has been observed by Werner (1993).

The technique enables the surgeon to estimate the depth of tumor penetration, to visualize the deep borders of the cancer to identify the relationship of the tumor to adjacent structures such as cartilage or soft tissues of the neck, and individually to adjust the safety margin so that the tumor is resected completely.

Individual Custom-Tailored Surgery (Taylor-Made Surgery), i.e., Individually Adapted Resection Margins

The *surgical strategy* is not only determined by preoperative findings, but the transoral resection rather follows the *individual spread* of the tumor as seen under the microscope. The concept of "custom-tailored surgery" means adjusting the surgical procedure individually to the intraoperative findings. This not only results in an oncologically sound resection of the tumor but also maximizes the possible *preservation of organ structures and function.*

The principle is to minimize the surgical morbidity while not compromising time-honored oncological principles (i.e., *less surgical radicality without loss of oncological radicality*).

Free Options for any Kind of Surgery

All surgical options are kept open during and after laser surgery. During the operation, the procedure can be changed to an external approach at any time. Postoperatively, further resections can be performed transorally with the laser, or a conventional partial or total resection can be carried out.

Laser Surgery can be Repeated at any Time

Laser surgery can be applied repeatedly at any stage for the treatment of local recurrences or second primaries.

Integration into any Therapeutic Concept

Adjuvant radiotherapy with or without chemotherapy may be started as soon as 2 weeks after a laser resection. The surgery actually results in an increase in blood flow and vascularization in the area of the primary tumor and the entire neck region. This constitutes particularly *favorable conditions* for subsequent irradiation and/or chemotherapy and increases their efficacy.

No reconstructive Surgery Necessary

The resulting defect after laser-surgical removal is not covered and no reconstructive surgery, for example using muscle flaps, is required. After spontaneous healing, the functional results are better and the chances for early detection of local recurrence are improved.

Low Perioperative Morbidity and Complication Rate

Tracheotomy is only rarely indicated, even after large resections. Secondary laryngectomy for functional reasons, for example persisting severe aspiration, has only been necessary very rarely. Considering the large open wound, postoperative secondary hemorrhage necessitating active intervention is less common than after conventional resections. There is little edema formation and wound healing is very satisfactory even when large areas of cartilage are exposed or resected. Only rarely have we encountered perichondritis or cartilage necrosis even in patients that underwent preoperative or postoperative irradiation, Laser treatment might have a lasting sterilizing and antibacterial effect. Patients usually experience very little or even no pain postoperatively.

Further Advantages

Length of operation, hospital stay, and duration of illness are markedly *shortened. Costs* are reduced accordingly. Last, but not least, *reintegration* of the patient and his *work* and *social life* is faster and more complete.

Immunology factors (Wustrow, 1995) are improved, and, although hard to prove, the psychological aspects without doubt play an integral role in oncological practice. Both are believed to have the ability to positively influence healing and function as well as the oncological results.

Disadvantages and Risks of Transoral Laser Surgery

The exposure of the operative field can be compromised by abnormal anatomical situations or unfavorable localization and extent of the tumor. Difficulties can arise in cases of tumor involvement of trachea and subglottis, deep infiltration of the tongue base, or tumor growth in the transitional area between hypopharynx and esophagus with invasion of the paraesophageal space. Such situations can prevent a curative resection.

Transoral procedures require a lot of *experience* in the various techniques of endoscopic microsurgery. The assessment of big lesions is only possible by combining several views of the different parts of the tumor to an overall impression in a mosaic-like fashion. This procedure is unfamiliar to many surgeons. A risk for the patient might arise from the incomplete resection by an inexperienced surgeon. The danger of accidental injury to the larger vessels is also increased when the surgeon lacks experience with endoscopic and conventional surgical techniques.

The limits of specimen processing and histological diagnosis are reached in the resection of more extensive tumors, as the orientation of the specimen and the correlation of clinical and pathological findings become increasingly difficult. The responsibility for a resection with clear margins lies primarily with the surgeon in this and any other type of surgery.

The surgeon performing conventional cancer surgery may be lulled into a false sense of security by handing the pathologist the specimen of the en bloc resection. Their high expectations for a definitive comment by the pathologist on tumor extent and the resection margins can often not be met. The various reasons for this have been discussed above. The greatest risk for the patient is, however, *undertreatment* due to inadequate experience of the surgeon or due to rating functional aspects higher than oncological principles.

Prerequisites for the Successful Use of Transoral Laser Microsurgery

A number of conditions have to be met to be able to perform oncologically sound transoral laser cancer surgery that also preserves function:

- A clear exposure of the region affected by the tumor must be obtained to allow the resection with clear margins all around the lesion. Optimal exposure requires appropriate experience of the surgeon. Knowledge of conventional surgical principles and techniques are a distinct advantage.
- A close cooperation with the pathologist is essential for minimally invasive surgery. The involved pathologist should be familiar with the special concerns and problems of this surgical approach. The complete resection of the tumor can be confirmed intraoperatively by frozen-section examination. Yet it is still mandatory to perform a postoperative systematic examination of the resected tumor bulk and the specimens obtained from the margins.
- Patients must be cooperative and motivated. This includes counseling on their disease and the envisaged stepwise procedure or "tailor-made surgery." Patients must also be prepared to change their habits and willing to attend the regular and close follow-up visits. Both contribute decisively to the success of the treatment.

Up-to-date Management Policy

Any tumor for which a curative procedure with preservation of function seems feasible is treated primarily with a transoral laser-surgical technique under the operating microscope. Concurrent surgical treatment of the neck, whether unilateral or bilateral, is dependent on the pretherapeutic status of the cervical lymph nodes, on the localization of the primary tumor (vocal cord vs. pyriform sinus), and on the final histology (grading G2 vs. G4 and depth of infiltration 3 mm vs. 7 mm). Our approach toward the neck is stepwise, as it is toward the primary tumor. This means that the intraoperative findings (with or without frozen-section diagnosis) are considered when deciding if further cervical levels have to be included in the selective neck dissection. The dissection method is always in accordance with the surgical principles for the classical functional neck dissection as described by Suarez. (Ambosch et al. 1996, Bocca et al. 1984, Byers et al. 1988, Manni v. d. Hoogen 1991, Medina, Byers 1989, Pelliteri 1997, Pitman 1997, Spiro et al. 1993, Spriano et al. 1998, Steiner 1984.)

However, we modify the technique by dissecting the relevant regions of the neck only from in front of the sternocleidomastoid muscle (Fig. 3.**6**). Even in cases of advanced metastatic disease in the neck, we strive for preservation of function during the dissection. The local integrity of the neck is largely preserved by limiting the functional neck dissection to the cervical levels that are preferred metastatic sites (levels I to VI) (Robbins et al, 1991) for the respective primary tumor. A careful surgical technique is employed and aims at preserving muscles, vessels, and nerves.

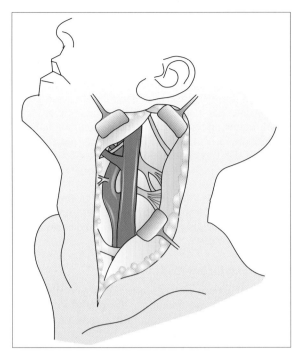

Fig. 3.**6** Schematic drawing of a selective neck dissection. The levels II and III are, for instance, resected in a patient with a larynx carcinoma and an N0 neck. The internal jugular vein, accessory nerve, and sternocleidomastoid muscle are spared in the process. The resection resembles a functional neck dissection but is limited to the two levels for which there is a high probability of clinically occult metastatic disease.

Since the early 1980s a selective neck dissection is routinely performed for N0–N2 necks. The oncological results are very satisfactory, similar to those after (modified) radical neck dissection. Side effects and complications are fewer and the functional and esthetic results clearly superior.

Timing of Neck Dissection

We usually perform the neck dissection after an interval of 4–8 days when the final histological report of the resected primary tumor is available. If necessary, a further resection of the primary tumor can then be performed in the same setting. An elective neck dissection (N0 neck) can be performed as late as 4–6 weeks after surgery for the primary tumor. It can then be combined with a revision of the site of the primary, and laser biopsies can be taken, particularly in patients that had extensive resections. In the rare cases, where the transoral resection has to be combined with an external approach, due to extensive infiltration of the soft tissues of the neck, the neck dissection is obviously performed at the same time. Another special situation is the resection of tumors of the lateral pharyngeal wall that have invaded the proximity of the vascular bundle in the neck. To prevent a through and through defect with potential fistula formation, the neck is operated not before 8 days after the transoral procedure. In the neck which is clinically free of metastases, this may even be delayed for 4–6 weeks.

In our experience there are a number of advantages in performing the resection of the primary tumor and the neck dissection in stages. The patient recovers faster and more completely. Functional rehabilitation, especially swallowing, is improved. Following extensive partial resections of larynx and pharynx without tracheotomy, transient aspiration can lead to severe coughing spells. This increases the danger of more or less serious hemorrhages in the neck if it has been operated on at the same time. Although the resulting hematomas can resorb, the functional and esthetic results are certainly better if bleeding under the flaps is altogether avoided. The main argument to delay the neck dissection is a biological consideration. This is largely based on the hypothesis of in-transit metastases. Although this has not been proved, theoretically these metastatic cells are then removed during the neck dissection.

Additional Therapy (Radiotherapy and/or Chemotherapy)

Any adjuvant treatment is primarily based on the intraoperative and pathological findings. Tumor site and extent play a role as do postoperative histological grading, typing, and staging of primary and cervical disease (pT, pN). Additional therapy for the primary tumor is, in our opinion, only indicated if it cannot be removed completely despite further attempts at resection and the remaining alternative is a radical operation (laryngopharyngectomy or glossectomy). Our criteria for adjuvant therapy on the basis of cervical metastases are: extracapsular spread, infiltration of lymph vessels, two or more lymph nodes involved, or a large solitary metastasis (pN2/3).

Laser Microsurgery for Laryngeal Carcinoma

Glottic Carcinomas
Carcinoma in situ, Microcarcinoma

Preoperative and Intraoperative Diagnosis

Diagnosis

Laryngeal carcinoma is usually suspected when a circumscribed area of mucosal change, for example leukoplakia, is discovered, commonly in the middle of the mobile part of the vocal cord, on the free edge of the cord. The clinical impression is confirmed by cytological diagnosis (PAP IV, V). Suspicion of carcinoma in situ, microinvasion, or frank carcinoma (microcarcinoma) is confirmed histologically by a biopsy specimen.

Diagnostic Procedure

In the awake patient (if necessary under topical anesthesia):
• Indirect laryngoscopy, endoscopy (90° telescope), or flexible endoscopy
– video stroboscopy
– voice analysis
– documentation for the patient's file and the oncological records (photos or reprints can always be made from the video recording) cytological smear.

Under general anesthesia during microlaryngoscopy:
• Laryngotracheobronchoscopy
– esophagoscopy
– microlaryngoscopic excision with the CO_2 laser.

The diagnostic procedure follows the routine laid out in Chapter 3, p. 33. The main indications are confirmed laryngeal carcinoma, patients with risk factors (smokers), and certain symptoms suggestive of more serious disease. We prefer to perform the transoral microsurgical treatment of laryngeal carcinoma under general anesthesia with endotracheal intubation (see Chapter 1, p. 2 and Chapter 4, p. 118 ff.).

Surgical Procedure for Circumscribed Early Lesions of the Midcord (pTis, pT1a; Fig. 3.7)
Diagnostic/Therapeutic Excision vs. Curative Resection

In cases with *negative* cytological or histological results, a diagnostic/therapeutic excision is indicated. This consists of a complete removal of all macroscopic disease

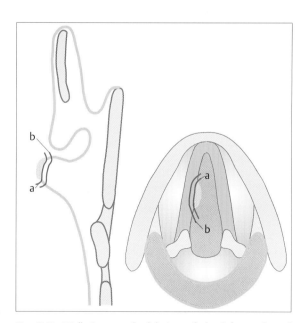

Fig. 3.**7** Well-circumscribed lesion of the left vocal cord suspicious of carcinoma. In the case of an excisional biopsy, only the lesion itself is excised (**a**). If there is a great suspicion of carcinoma (cytological result PAP IV or PAP V) or if a previous biopsy confirmed a malignancy, a curative resection is performed with an individually selected resection margin of 1–3 mm (**b** and **c**).

in the form of an excisional biopsy. In cases of a *positive* cytology, or biopsy-proved carcinoma similarly an excision biopsy is performed, this time with the advantage of hindsight. The entire lesion is excised with an appropriate resection margin.

Account is taken of the individual circumstances of each patient, but the aim in all cases is to perform an adequate *excision* biopsy. The aim is to avoid a second general anesthetic and the associated risks to an elderly patient, which would become necessary if the final histological result shows positive margins. Although this occurs in less than 5% of our patients, it is a factor that must be considered in the individual patient with a high anesthetic risk.

Operative Procedure

The use of an acuspot or microspot control results in minimal char formation and is particularly suitable for this application, as it is for benign lesions of the vocal folds. Continuous super pulse and low power settings (Chapter 1, p. 10) have given us very satisfactory results. The histological assessment of the resection margins was facilitated by this technique, despite relatively close margins. The average distance between tumor and line of resection was 1.5 mm on the basal aspects. The vocal function was in general almost normal after such limited excisional biopsies.

If the surgeon has not had much experience with the laser, the resection line can first be outlined by small marks made with the laser. These dots can then be connected by laser cuts. It is advisable to set the laser on the "interval" rather than the "continuous" mode. The laser gives off single impulses in this mode and the surgeon has more time to perform an accurate cut.

Laser excision vs. excision with conventional instruments. The first-generation CO_2 lasers produced a notably wider line of carbonization. While using this early equipment, we found that the smaller the lesion of the cord and the more obscure its pathology, the less suited the laser was as a surgical instrument. In principle small, well-circumscribed lesions can be resected safely and with good preservation of function (voice sparing) even without the laser (Kleinsasser, 1988).

✍ The use of modern lasers that allow dissection almost without carbonization have the following advantages:
- There is almost always a bloodless field, resulting in high surgical precision and providing excellent conditions for the intraoperative assessment of the tissues,
- Hemostasis in the form of conventional electrocautery is not necessary. Tissue is spared and a better functional result achieved.

Unexpected invasion of the musculature by the tumor. The findings on stroboscopy, microscopic impression, and palpation (testing of the mobility of the tumor carrying mucosa over the vocal ligament) give valuable hints and usually a superficial tumor can be differentiated from a deeply infiltrating cancer on clinical grounds.

If tumor is encountered in the submucosal space during oncological excision of a superficial lesion, the resection must be made wider in order to guarantee an adequate safety margin.

Securing an Adequate Resection Margin

There are a number of ways to achieve this goal:
- The *frozen-section examination of the excised tissue* provides a certain reassurance. Since the processing of the material does not imply the systematic examination of all margins, an absolutely certain answer cannot be provided.
- *Punch biopsies* from the wound edges, especially from the deep resection margin (musculature). We reject these random biopsies, as they are not representative of the whole area of resection. They can thus provide false negative results.
- *Further resection* in the depth of the wound. A representative excision biopsy is obtained from the entire wound surface either with conventional instruments or the laser (microspot or acuspot). Frozen-section examination is possible, but again an absolutely reliable answer must not be expected. This technique provides maximum reliability, unfortunately, however, at the expense of additional tissue, which is sacrificed in the process (voice quality).
- No additional tissue is resected immediately, but the *definitive histological result is awaited.* If necessary, an additional resection is performed at this later stage (in our patient population this occurs in less than 5% of cases). With increasing experience, these additional resections become less and less common.

In patients with a high anesthetic risk, both patient and surgeon would rather avoid a second general anesthesia. We usually choose a wider resection margin in these cases to avoid any additional procedure. Alternatively, extra tissue can be resected and submitted for an intraoperative frozen section to confirm a clear margin. Tumors in patients who are professional voice users, or those who are particularly concerned with a good postoperative voice function, are resected with a narrow margin. We await the histological result and put up with the possibility of an additional resection during a second microlaryngoscopy. In our experience patients often opt for this stepwise approach after an intensive counseling session before the operation. The problems and the chance of more than one operation are explained to the patient as are the advantageous preservation of tissue and functional aspects.

Previously Biopsied Carcinomas

We prefer smear cytology obtained under endoscopic control for the diagnosis of small glottic carcinomas. A sample can also be sent for microbiological examination when tuberculosis is suspected. Alternatively, the lesion, for example a leukoplakia, can be excised completely without an initial cytological diagnosis. In our experience punch biopsies are only random samples of a lesion and can be unrepresentative. It is therefore best if patients with the suspicion of laryngeal carcinoma are sent to a larger referral center. Diagnostic procedures of any kind should then be performed at this institution, where the patient also receives the definitive treatment. It can of course happen that a lesion that appears benign or premalignant, proves to be an invasive carcinoma on histology after the microlaryngoscopic excision has been performed.

The disadvantage with glottic tumors that have been previously biopsied is that the *discrimination between tumor and healthy tissue* becomes more difficult during endoscopic excision (Fig. 3.**8**). Inflammatory and reparative processes following the initial surgery lead to the formation of granulation tissue, which may be confused with the carcinoma. The results of microscopic surgery under these circumstances are likely to be less than satisfactory, as either too much or too little tissue may be excised. Unnecessary excision of the vocal ligament would, for instance, lead to a poor postoperative voice, too conservative excision to local recurrence.

Preparation of the Excision
Biopsy for Histological Examination

The specimen that has been obtained through the microlaryngoscopic excision must be carefully laid out and marked by the surgeon. This helps the pathologist with orientation and subsequent examination of the resected tissue and is a prerequisite for a reliable histopathological assessment of lateral and deep excision margins. After the deep surface of the resection has been marked with a pen, the specimen is pinned onto a piece of cork or paper and labeled with "anterior" and "posterior" (Fig. 3.**9**).

Histological Processing and Evaluation

The histological work-up of a specimen excised from the vocal cord follows the guidelines described by Kleinsasser and Glanz (1984). The pathologist performs serial sections through the tissue. At the Institute of Pathology at the University of Göttingen, Germany, 2-mm intervals are chosen (Fig. 3.**10** and 3.**11**).

Difficulties with the histological interpretation only arise from very close margins. An example of a well-demarcated carcinoma of the glottis is shown in

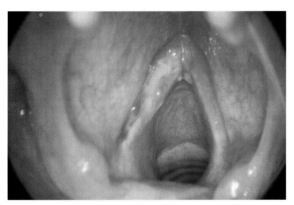

a

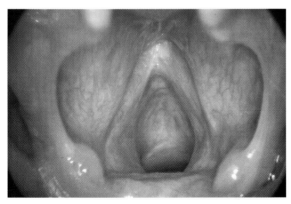

b

Fig. 3.**8** Glottic carcinoma (T1a) before and after laser resection (endoscopic view, 90° telescope). **a** Preoperative finding after multiple biopsies had been taken at another hospital. The tumor reaches onto the anterior commissure. It is difficult to distinguish between reactive, inflammatory granulation tissue and tumor tissue. **b** A good functional result was achieved after laser resection of the lesion, which included the anterior commissure.

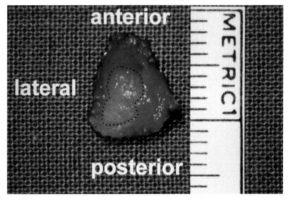

Fig. 3.**9** Glottic carcinoma (T1). The specimen has been obtained by en bloc resection. In order to help the pathologist with the orientation and the processing of the specimen, it is labelled appropriately and pinned onto a piece of paper or cork.

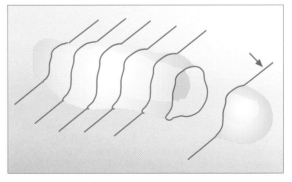

Fig. 3.**10** Microcarcinoma of the vocal fold. The excision specimen from the glottis is processed by serial sectioning.

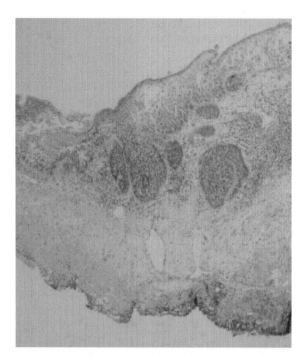

Fig. 3.**11**   Histological section through a squamous cell carcinoma of the vocal cord (hematoxylin-eosin stain). The basal margin is free of tumor. The distance between tumor and basal resection margin is 0.5 mm; the zone of carbonization is 50 mm wide.

Fig. 3.**12**. Three different lines of resection (a–c) are depicted together with their respective safety margins. The corresponding histological sections are shown for comparison:

– Resection line a reaches onto tumor and thus there is a positive margin; an additional resection is indicated (Fig. 3.**12a**).
– Resection b has a narrow margin of healthy tissue (Fig. 3.**12b**).
– An excessively wide margin of normal tissue was taken in c(Fig. 3.**12c**).

The histological situation has consequences for the follow-up treatment.

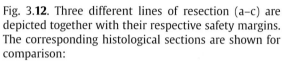

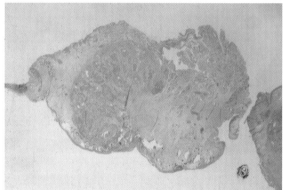

a

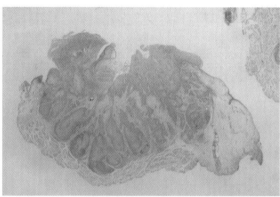

b

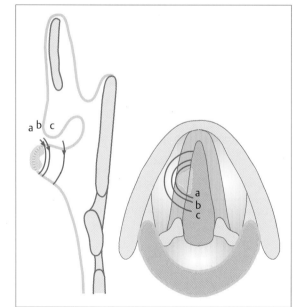

Fig. 3.**12**   Different safety margins for an early glottic carcinoma. The respective resection lines are indicated (**a–c**). **a** Tumor reaches onto the line of resection. **b** Close distance between tumor and resection line. The tumor is, however, resected well within normal tissue. **c** Wide safety margin around the superficial tumor. The corresponding histological sections are shown in photos **a–c**.

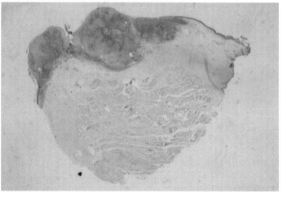

c

Deduction from the Histological Report

The laryngologist has to respond to the following factors:
- Intraoperative findings,
- Histological diagnosis and comments on the resection margins,
- Postoperative course.

On the basis of this deliberation, the surgeon decides on the further management. The patient should be counseled again at this stage and informed about the situation and the further plans. Possible alternatives might be the necessity for immediate additional resection, close follow-up or follow-up visits at longer intervals, etc.

Examples of two unequivocal situations are:
- The histology report shows tumor-free margins according to resection line c (Fig. 3.**12**). This lesion has clearly been *completely excised.* Consequently, initial close follow-up by the referring otorhinolaryngologist and 3-monthly check-ups by the treating oncology clinic are adequate. Two visits to the cancer surgeon in the second postoperative year and from there on yearly visits are sufficient.
- *Tumor has been cut through* (resection line a, Fig. 3.**12**) and residual cancer left behind. In this situation an additional resection is definitely indicated.

The decision becomes more difficult when the pathologist expresses doubts about the completeness of the resection or reports a very narrow margin (resection line b, Fig. 3.**12**). An individualized answer must be found to the question of whether immediate additional resections should be performed or whether a close follow-up consisting of laryngoscopy, smears for cytology, and stroboscopy for the early diagnosis of submucous recurrence is to be preferred. The patient's desire for oncological safety rather than good voice function plays a significant role. A number of other factors should also be considered:

Intraoperative Factors

The specimen examined by the pathologist might not be representative of the actual extent of the resection for the following reasons:
- Heat artifact over a thin zone on the resection margin. This may make the pathological interpretation of a clear margin difficult.
- There may have been more tissue excised than is evident to the pathologist due to the following reasons:
- Using a laser with a large spot-size and consequently vaporizing a broad band of tissue.
- Coagulating small bleeding points on the wound surface with the laser or smoothening of the wound surface by laser evaporation of tissue.

Therefore, it is not surprising that in some cases the pathologist reports tumor up to the margin of the specimen but that in the additional tissue resected from the particular area no tumor can be detected.

Quality of Histological Work-Up and Examination

The amount of time and effort spent by the pathologist on the specimens is of great importance. The number of sections taken from the specimen is decisive, as is the sectioning technique to avoid artifacts. Correct handling will thus eliminate pitfalls that can result in a wrong interpretation of the specimen. The experience of the pathologist is obviously of paramount importance.

Postoperative Course

The patient's willingness and ability to cooperate in a postoperative program of close follow-ups must be considered in the decision between "immediate additional resection" and a "wait and see" policy. This is of even greater importance in cases of doubtful or very narrow margins. *Patient cooperation* is a basic requirement for the strategy of close follow-up, since this puts more strain on the patient. Apart from the time that he has to put aside, the patient has to undergo laryngoscopy, smears for cytology, stroboscopy, and video documentation. There are patients who opt for an additional resection sooner rather than later after their postoperative counseling session. Other patients attach more value to an almost normal functioning voice and are prepared to accept the small risk and the greater postoperative strain put on them. A favorable aspect is the fact that residual or recurrent tumor in the area of the vocal cord can usually be detected at an early stage.

Recurrent tumor growth on the surface can commonly be recognized by the formation of hyperplastic tissue or conspicuous scar tissue (Fig. 3.**14c**). If the operated vocal cord shows reduced mobility on stroboscopic examination or, more significantly, with indirect or endoscopy (90° telescope), recurrent submucosal tumor growth must be suspected. A microlaryngoscopic examination and excision biopsy must be performed preferably after cytology of a laryngeal smear. Patients who do not attend the follow-up and will not even attend a private otorhinolaryngology surgeon or the treating oncology unit despite worsening voice problems, run the risk of tumor progression. The chance for an oncologically sound removal of the recurrent tumor and simultaneous preservation of function becomes progressively smaller in these cases.

Further Treatment and After Care

Guidelines for the Patient

The patient is requested to attend his otorhinolaryngologist for an assessment after discharge from the hospital. A follow-up visit is usually scheduled for 4–6 weeks after the procedure. After the excision of a small glottic carcinoma, usually neither topical nor systemic treatment in the form of cortisone, anti-inflammatory, or antibiotics is necessary. Inhalation therapy is only of restricted value for a small wound on the vocal cord.

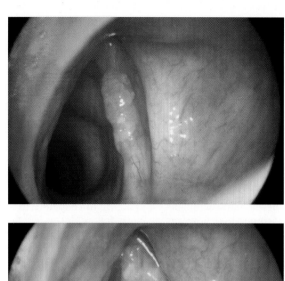

a

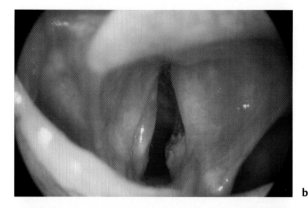

b

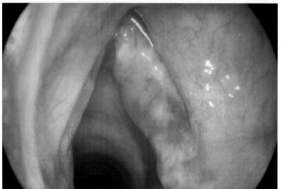

c

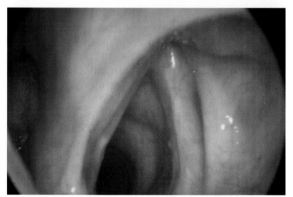

d

Fig. 3.**13**   Glottic carcinoma of the free edge of the mobile right vocal fold (T1a). The patient's course has been documented endoscopically (90° telescope). **a** Preoperative view. **b** Four hours after surgery. The wound defect can be seen with traces of carbonized tissue (operation in 1979).

c Wound healing takes place with marked fibrin production and the formation of granulation tissue. **d** The final condition of the right vocal fold after wound healing has been completed. A discrete scar is visible.

Voice rest is, however, important and the advice is similar to that after resection of benign lesions in phonosurgery. Depending on the patient's occupation, this entails sick leave of a few weeks.

⚐ Smoking is prohibited under all circumstances, and alcohol should be reduced to an absolute minimum. The inhalation of irritant gasses or fumes at the workplace must be avoided.

Wound Healing

During the healing process, a more or less marked formation of fibrinous membranes and granulation tissue occurs on the wound surface (Fig. 3.**13c**, 3.**18b**). There are also patients who have a particularly strong tendency toward the formation of granulation tissue. An exceptionally strong inflammatory response in and around the wound can be the cause for this, as can undue strain on the voice. Surgical removal should only take place for *granulation tissue that persists* for more than 6–12 weeks and if significant problems with the voice are encountered (Fig. 3.**14b**).

☝ Persistent granulation tissue can be ablated in the chair under endoscopic (90° telescope) control after application of a topical anesthetic.

⚡ In professional voice users it is, however, recommended that the granulations be removed at microlaryngoscopy.

An *atypical scar formation* can occur. By this is meant a spindle-shaped swelling of the vocal cord which can appear as hyperplasia in the area of the resection (Fig. 3.**14c**). It must always raise the suspicion of residual tumor. Similar to the formation of keloid in the skin, some patients have a tendency for the formation of hypertrophic scar tissue in wounds of the mucosa.

Diagnostic procedure: Stroboscopy under magnification should be performed and a smear obtained for cytology. The area is finally excised with the laser under microscopic control. These measures help to clarify the underlying pathology and at the same time improve the voice. A laser excision is especially indicated in those cases where the tumor had been resected with a very narrow margin.

Any *new tissue formation,* such as hyperplasia, leukoplakia, papilloma, etc., must be excised. This also applies to a unilateral inflammation of the vocal cord which persists for months after the excision of an early-stage tumor (Fig. 3.**14c**). Follow-up examinations with stroboscopy are especially important in these cases.

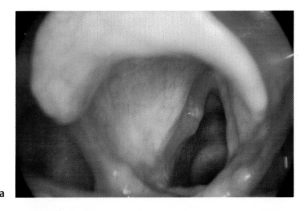

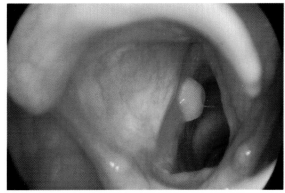

a

b

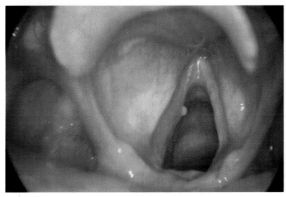

c

Fig. 3.14 Residual tumor after laser surgery. **a** Glottic carcinoma on the left after a biopsy had been taken at another institution. **b** Four weeks after laser excision. There is erythema of the vocal fold and mushrooming granulation tissue. This was removed under topical anesthesia endoscopic (90° telescope) and the histological examination showed no malignancy in the resected specimen. **c** After another 6 weeks a spindle-shaped swelling of the left vocal fold with a small area of granulation tissue became manifest. Together with the atypical scar formation, this raised the suspicion of residual tumor, which was proved cytologically and also histologically after a second curative procedure.

Speech Therapy After Complete Healing

Wound healing is usually complete after 3–4 weeks. The first follow-up examination by the surgeon, including a phoniatric assessment, is scheduled for 4–6 weeks following the surgery. During this visit, it is decided whether further speech therapy will be necessary. The following factors are taken into consideration:

– Findings at laryngoscopy and glottic function (stroboscopy and voice analysis),
– Age of patient,
– Occupation,
– Patient's preferences.

Postoperative Care

The patient should be followed up at short intervals by his referring otorhinolaryngologist and at longer intervals at the treating oncology center, preferably by the surgeon who performed the operation. We generally recommend a second examination after 6–8 weeks and afterward at 3-monthly intervals for the first year. The routine patients are then followed up three times in the second year, twice in the third year, and at yearly intervals from the fourth year onward.

Often, however, an *individualized* plan is drawn up for the postoperative care. A number of individual factors related to tumor, patient, and therapy thereby determine the frequency, type, and extent of the follow-up visits. The *individual risk of a residual tumor or a second primary* is a crucial factor in the planning

of the aftercare. The probability of complete tumor resection is taken into consideration. Factors like the patient's exposure to carcinogenic substances such as tobacco smoke and excessive amounts of alcohol play a decisive role.

Finally, the age of the patient must be considered in devising an aftercare strategy. A frail 85-year-old patient with a completely resected T1 glottic tumor who possibly lives far from the center will obviously not be followed up in 4-weekly intervals. Although general guidelines can be given for the intervals of follow-up visits, the treating physician should always find an individual strategy, based on the above-mentioned criteria.

"Large" T1a Glottic Tumor (with or without Anterior Commissure or Vocal Process Involvement)

Procedure

The decision whether the tumor is resected in two or three pieces, i.e., whether one or two incisions have to be made through the tumor, is based on the surface extension of the tumor and its suspected depth of infiltration. Preoperative diagnostic aids and the intraoperative incision through the tumor help with this decision. In a clearly superficial lesion which does not cover the entire cord and infiltrates to a depth of only approximately 2 mm, i.e., a microcarcinoma, a single incision through the middle of the tumor is sufficient to estimate

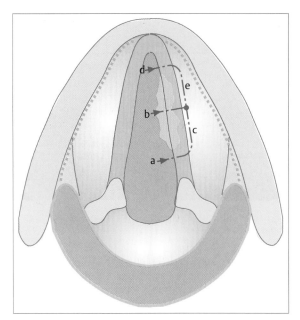

Fig. 3.**15**   Right-sided glottic carcinoma. The resection is performed in two pieces. The first incision (**a**) is made posteriorly through healthy tissue with an adequate safety margin. The second cut goes through the middle of the tumor (**b**). The tumor borders can be seen on the cut surface (see Fig. 3.**16**). A margin of 1–3 mm is chosen for the resection and the first specimen is obtained by freeing the tumor laterally (**c**). Following this the anterior resection is performed with a margin of healthy tissue (**d**) and the operation completed by lateral resection of the remaining tumor (**e**).

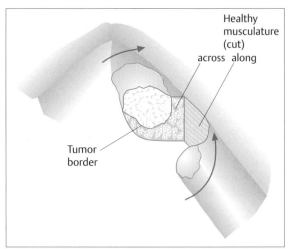

Fig. 3.**16**   This drawing shows the cut surface after a cut has been made through the carcinoma of the right vocal fold (T1). This allows the direct inspection of the depth of infiltration of the carcinoma and of the surrounding healthy structures (musculature).

the actual depth of infiltration. The subsequent laser surgical treatment is the same as for small, well-circumscribed lesions.

Fig. 3.**15** shows a graphic impression of the resection lines for a tumor with a depth of infiltration of 3 mm. The resection starts posteriorly within healthy tissue (resection line a) and is followed by an incision through the middle of the tumor (line b). The first specimen consisting of the posterior tumor mass is obtained by dissecting laterally and inferiorly (resection line c). The next step is the anterior incision through normal tissue (line d), after which the resection is completed by freeing the tumor anterolaterally (line e).

Resection Margins

Deep resection. The border between tumor and surrounding normal tissue is identified on the cut surface (Fig. 3.**16**). An individually appropriate safety margin of 1–3 mm is then selected. This lateral area of resection within the musculature is again marked with blue ink on the resected specimen. It is commonly referred to as the deep resection margin by the pathologists.

Anterior and posterior resection. On the mucosal surface we choose a safety margin of 1–2 mm. The specimen is pinned onto a piece of paper and appropriately labelled (Fig. 3.**9**.). This helps in the processing

and the serial sectioning of the specimen and allows the objective histological diagnosis of a complete resection with negative margins to be made.

If the tumor has not yet quite reached the anterior commissure, the resection line can be taken exactly through the anterior commissure, albeit with a narrower margin. The formation of a web is thus usually prevented (Fig. 3.**17** and 3.**18**). The same applies to tumors that have reached the area of the vocal process. One dissects closely in front of the arytenoid cartilage and, if necessary, includes the vocal process in the resection. If the tumor reaches the anterior commissure, a small tumor-free portion of the anterior contralateral cord must also be included in the resection. This will of necessity result in a web of the anterior commissure (Fig. 5.**4**).

Alternatively, the resection can be performed in the following manner: The tumor is initially resected with relatively narrow margins, after which *additional slices of tissue* of 1–2 mm thickness are obtained from the lateral (basal), anterior, and posterior wound surfaces (Fig. 3.**19**). Further slices can similarly be resected from the superior (sinus of Morgagni) and the inferior mucosal margins of the vocal fold. These additional specimens are then submitted to the pathologist for histological examination to determine whether carcinoma is present in them. Single nests of tumor cells are thereby distinguished from clear infiltration by tumor. If these specimens are not meticulously marked immediately after the resection, it becomes impossible for the pathologist to comment on their exact topographical orientation.

Additional loss of functionally important structures is the price that is to be paid for this high demand for oncological safety and the unwillingness to take a small

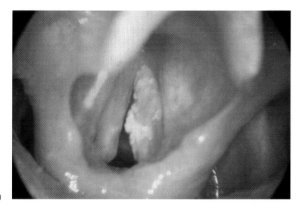

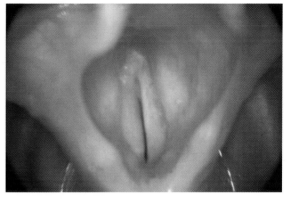

Fig. 3.**17** Glottic carcinoma (T1a) before and after laser surgical treatment (endoscopic view, 90° telescope). **a** Pre-operative finding: white keratotic cover of almost the entire right vocal fold. The vocal process has been partially involved and the lesion has reached the anterior commissure. **b** After laser resection of the carcinoma, which did not infiltrate deeply. A complete closure of the glottis is achieved during phonation, which resulted in an excellent voice quality.

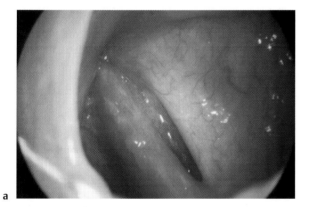

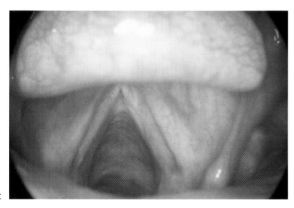

Fig. 3.**18** Recurrence of a glottic carcinoma (anterior and middle third of right vocal fold) after failure of irradiation treatment before and after laser resection (endoscopic view, 90° telescope). **a** Preoperative findings of irregularly shaped neoplasm of the anterior and middle third of the right vocal fold. A biopsy of the lesion confirmed the presence of a carcinoma. **b** The formation of fibrin and granulation tissue in the area of the resection can be clearly seen 1 week after laser resection. **c** Final result after wound healing has been accomplished. Despite the intermittent formation of granulation tissue, a very satisfactory result has been achieved also from a functional point of view.

risk. Both surgeon and patient must be aware of this. We do not perform these additional resections as a general safety precaution. However, this technique is resorted to in the rare cases where intraoperatively the suspicion of incomplete resection is raised.

If *tumor is found in the specimen*, the pathologist is required to comment on the grade of differentiation, depth of infiltration, and the involvement of the basal resection margin.

Our principal concern with all specimens submitted to the pathologist is the *basal resection margin*. The resection margins on the mucosal surface leaves the surgeon with much greater confidence due to the high magnification of the microscope, especially when an adequate margin is kept.

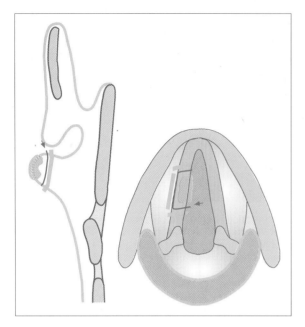

Fig. 3.**19**   Left glottic carcinoma (T1) without involvement of anterior commissure or vocal process. A laser excision is performed with further specimens (anterior, lateral, posterior, superior, and inferior) obtained immediately during the primary surgery. These additional specimens taken after a marginal excision of an early glottic carcinoma must be histologically free of tumor. We usually avoid these extra resections since too much functionally important tissue is sacrificed in the process. Adequate microsurgical experience allows the intraoperative distinction between tumor and normal tissue to be made with great certainty in the previously untreated vocal cord. In our experience it is therefore sufficient to keep a distance of 1–3 mm, to meticulously mark the basal resection margins with blue ink, and to perform a further resection in a second procedure if there was doubt about the initial margins. The average resection margin in our group of patients measures 1.5 mm on the histological specimens for these T1 lesions.

T1b Tumor of Both Vocal Cords (with or without Involvement of the Anterior Commissure)

Procedure

For carcinoma in situ or the rare carcinomas of both vocal folds *without* involvement of the anterior commissure the procedure is the same as it has been described for unilateral glottic carcinoma.

Carcinoma of Both Vocal Folds with Involvement of the Anterior Commissure (Fig. 3.20)

In cases of marginal involvement of the anterior commissure without subglottic extension, the anterior commissure is resected together with the bilateral cord lesion. The dissection is carried along the thyroid cartilage under high magnification of the operating microscope.

Intraoperative assessment. The side of the perichondrium facing the cartilage should be tumor-free. Again, the basal resection margin, i.e., the surface facing the thyroid cartilage is stained blue for improved orientation of the pathologist.

Another possibility is the transection of the tumor precisely through the anterior commissure in order to better judge the distance between tumor and perichondrium (Fig. 3.**21**). This technique is advocated for tumors that are not just small extensions across the anterior commissure onto the contralateral cord, but those with considerable subglottic or supraglottic extent.

Special Situation of an Exophytic Tumor Obstructing the Entire Anterior Glottis

Some tumors present as large, space-occupying lesions and the tendency to bleed easily even with the slightest manipulation. Difficulties can arise when one tries to find the base of these tumors and establish whether the tumor has its main origin on only *one* vocal cord or to what extent it involves the contralateral cord. Contralateral involvement may be simulated by an impression that a large exophytic tumor can leave on the contralateral vocal fold due to the close contact.

We use a special protector to obtain clarity and to help in the ensuing surgical procedure (Fig. 1.**6**). The protector is slowly advanced anteriorly along the cords. The uninvolved or less involved vocal fold is pushed laterally by the protector (Fig. 3.**22**). At the same time it may be helpful to pull the tumor laterally toward the other side with a small grasping forceps or a suction cannula. Rather strong suction is required for this purpose of retraction. With the protection of the contralateral cord guaranteed, a partial ablation of the exophytic lesion in the form of a debulking procedure can now take place (Fig. 3.**22**). After this rough reduction of tumor mass, the residual tumor can be removed as previously described. Medial retraction of the tissue containing the residual tumor is only possible after the debulking. It facilitates the identification of the lateral tumor borders, allows for unimpaired dissection and ensures that an adequate resection margin can be kept. In these cases the dissection almost always follows along the thyroid cartilage. In only few cases can connective tissue or muscle tissue be preserved in this area. The basal surface of the specimens from this resection are marked in the usual way and examined histologically.

Anterior Commissure – Risk Area and Origin of Local Recurrences

There are reports in the literature of very high recurrence rates for tumors involving the anterior commissure. Consequently, laser surgery of tumors of the anterior commissure and even lesions which barely reach the commissure have been discouraged. We have found a higher recurrence rate compared with midcordal lesions for tumors involving the anterior commissure. Local recurrences were observed especially in tumors

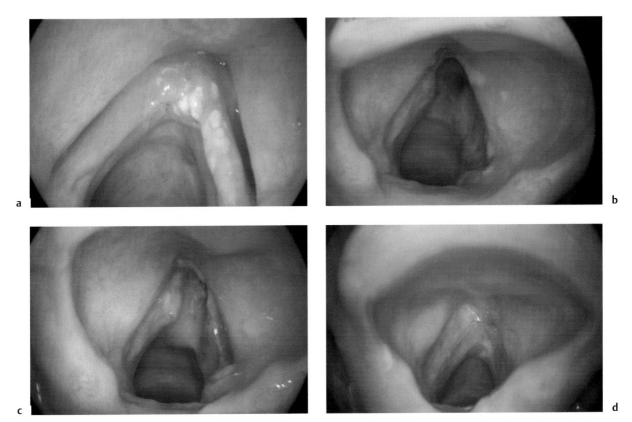

Fig. 3.**20** Glottic carcinoma with involvement of the anterior commissure (T1b) before and after laser resection. The course of the healing phase is shown. **a** Preoperative endoscopic photograph (90° telescope). Leukoplakia and keratotic foci on the anterior and middle parts of the right vocal cord. The anterior commissure and the left anterior vocal cord are involved by disease. Cytology result was PAP V; histology confirmed an infiltrating squamous cell carcinoma. **b** One week after the operation. The fibrinous layers were removed by swabbing with a cotton wool applicator one to two times per week. **c** The wound after 3 weeks. **d** The final result after completion of wound healing shows a web of the anterior glottis and a distinct loss of substance in the region of the right vocal cord.

with subglottic extension. The reason was, however, not a missed infiltration of the thyroid cartilage, which is rather rare in these tumors, but most probably the underestimation of the inferior and anterior tumor extent as these lesions were found to infiltrate or break through the cricothyroid membrane. Incomplete resection of tumor in this region occurred especially with en bloc resections and has resulted in the local recurrences. For this reason the surgical steps of resections in this difficult area of anterior glottis and subglottis are discussed in more detail.

Mistakes and Pitfalls of Resect of Anterior Commissure Carcinomas

As discussed above, the main reason for local recurrences in this area is insufficient radicality and thus an incomplete resection of the most anterior glottis and subglottis. An adequate exposure, which is not always possible, is the prerequisite for a safe resection of carcinomas in this region. A certain degree of courage is required from the surgeon to expose the thyroid cartilage and, if necessary, to remove parts of the cartilage and/or the cricothyroid ligament. A mistake which we made initially is the attempt to remove the tumor in one piece. This makes a complete resection of the tumor more difficult. In our experience the real depth of infiltration can only be recognized if the tumor is transected and the cut surface inspected intraoperatively. It is also the only way to see the true tumor borders and its relation to the surrounding structures, such as cartilage and cricothyroid membrane, and therefore a prerequisite to find the appropriate resection line. Otherwise, the infiltration of the thyroid cartilage, although this is a rare occurrence, might be missed. Kirchner (1989), in appraising his large series of serially sectioned larynges, paid special attention to the anterior commissure. He showed that the risk of infiltration of the thyroid cartilage by these carcinomas only existed in tumors with significant vertical extension. Of particular importance to us is the recognition of the subglottic spread toward or through the cricothyroid membrane.

⚡ During resection of the subglottic area, the surgeon can easily miss tumor that has grown around the inferior edge of the thyroid cartilage and broken

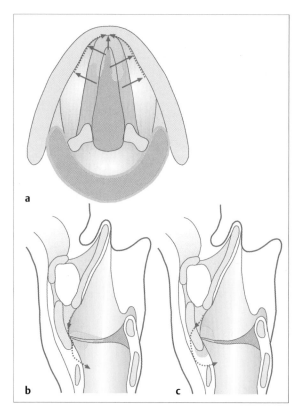

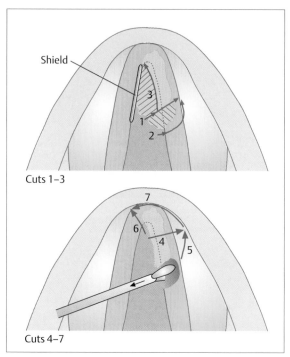

Fig. 3.**21**   Carcinoma of the anterior glottis and subglottis. In these cases there is a definite possibility of infiltration not only of the thyroid cartilage but even more so of the cricothyroid membrane. The resection of these tumors is performed in several pieces. **a** In the area of the anterior commissure a vertical incision should be made to enable the surgeon to directly see the deep tumor border on the cut surface and assess whether the soft tissues of the neck have been invaded. **b** After the anteroinferior dissection along the thyroid cartilage, parts of the cricothyroid membrane can be removed if this is deemed necessary. **c** The inferior aspect of the thyroid cartilage must be included in the resection if the tumor cannot be safely removed under microscopic vision due to more extensive infiltration of the soft tissues of the neck.

Fig. 3.**22**   Resection technique for an exophytic tumor of the anterior glottis. This tumor originates from the right vocal fold and involves the anterior commissure. First the posterior part of the tumor is resected (1, 2). Subsequently, the main bulk of the lesion is removed by amputating the exophytic component (3). A straight shield is used to protect the healthy left vocal fold. The exact extensions of the tumor in the anterior commissure become visible after the tumor has been debulked. The remaining tumor is mobilized medially and high magnification of the operating microscope is used to resect the anterior and lateral aspects of the tumor (4–7).

through the cricothyroid membrane. This error is more likely when using a laser that causes excessive carbonization during cutting. In our opinion the inadequate resection of this area is the main cause for local tumor recurrence.

In these cases of tumor escaping the confines of the larynx, we follow the tumor until it has been completely resected. Relatively extensive dissection of the prelaryngeal soft tissues and resection of the inferior parts of the thyroid cartilage may become necessary in the process. We recommend that surgeons who have little laser surgical experience should resort to an external approach in these cases of cartilage infiltration and extralaryngeal tumor spread. From a transcervical approach a frontolateral vertical partial laryngeal resection, including the anterior commissure, can be carried

out. Unfortunately, many laryngologists prefer irradiation therapy or a total laryngectomy in these borderline cases.

Strategy to Avoid Local Recurrences in the Anterior Commissure

1. The operation must be performed under high magnification and the resection is done in stepwise fashion. This allows for better recognition of the actual depth of infiltration and the topographical relations with perichondrium, cartilage, and cricothyroid membrane.
2. Careful histological assessment is made of the "stepped" specimens. If necessary, conventional instruments (e.g., round knife, elevator) need to be employed in the dissection around the thyroid cartilage. The tissue is stripped from the cartilage and the deep

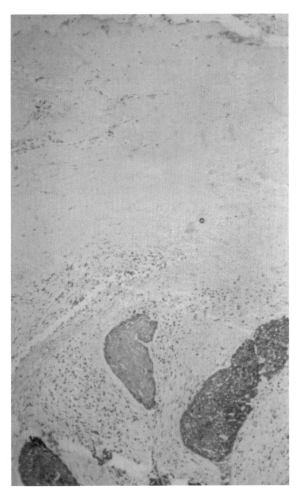

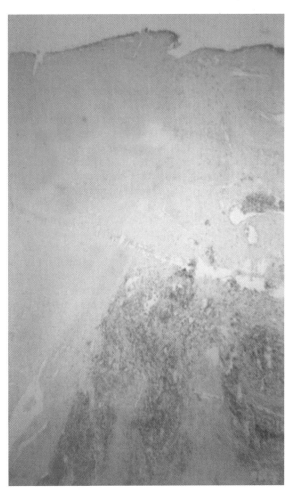

Fig. 3.**23** Carcinoma of the anterior glottis. This shows a section through the specimen from the anterior commissure (anticytokeratin stain). The finger-like tumor extensions come close to the connective tissue ("perichondrium"). The charred resection margin close to the thyroid cartilage is, however, tumor-free.

Fig. 3.**24** Carcinoma of the anterior glottis with infiltration of the connective tissue ("perichondrium"). This section is taken from the anterior commissure. The carcinoma can be seen to extend onto the thyroid cartilage, which has been included in the resection for reasons of oncological safety.

margin is marked blue. When the laser is used for the dissection, the tissue is retracted toward the lumen. Forceful retraction minimizes the carbonization of the deep resection surfaces (Fig. 3.**22** and 3.**23**). An intraoperative frozen-section examination of additional specimens from the margins is an option. These should obviously be free of tumor.

3. The line of resection must reach sufficiently far anteriorly and inferiorly into the subglottis and the tumor must be followed along its extensions. The borders of the carcinoma must be clearly defined and an adequate safety margin must be kept.

4. If there is suspicion of infiltration of the cartilage and/or the cricothyroid membrane, the suspicious looking areas are excised with the laser along their circumference until cartilage is reached. Conventional instruments are then used to "break out" the corresponding piece of cartilage for the subsequent histological examination (Fig. 3.**24**).

5. If the thyroid cartilage is clearly involved (infiltrated by tumor or clear tumor break-through) the resection has to be more liberal and follow a wider line. It can even become necessary to resect the inferior edge of the thyroid cartilage in order to gain access to the soft tissues of the neck. This is required for a complete resection of tumors that have eroded through the cricothyroid membrane (Fig. 3.**21**).

With limited experience in laser surgery it may become necessary to change to an external approach to ensure the complete resection of the tumor. This is necessary in particular for difficult local situations where a safe endoscopic removal of the tumor can no longer be guaranteed and for severe hemorrhages which cannot be controlled via the transoral route. It depends on the extent of the resection whether larynx and trachea can be closed primarily or whether a temporary larygo-tracheostomy is necessary. With adequate experience, tumors with erosion of the thyroid cartilage and infiltration of the soft tissues of the neck can be resected from a transoral approach. Complete resections of cancers can even be performed all the way into the subcutaneous tissue. However, it must be said that the safer method, especially for the less experienced surgeon, is the transcervical approach in these extreme situations of gross extralaryngeal tumor spread. This will help to avoid serious complications and make sure the resection of the tumor is complete. Larger hemorrhages from the thyroid gland can be difficult to control endoscopically. If the cricothyroid artery is encountered, a vascular clip must be used to achieve hemostasis.

Finally, it is not important whether the approach was transoral or transcervical, but whether a complete resection of the tumor could be achieved and a total laryngectomy avoided. In the particular case of anterior glottic carcinomas without involvement of cheostoma in situ after very extensive resections (especially operations for recurrence), where large parts of the thyroid cartilage have to be removed and the posterior resection extends up to the arytenoid cartilages. This epithelialized fistula is closed surgically in a second procedure.

6. Microlaryngoscopy is performed after 4–6 weeks for control purposes. Excisional biopsies should be taken liberally to exclude residual tumor.

Aftercare – Oncological and Functional Aspects

Microlaryngoscopic Assessment With Laser Biopsies

This examination is performed 4–6 weeks after the resection of very extensive tumors or if the completeness of the resection could not be proved histologically. Initially the granulation tissue is ablated. Deep biopsies are then taken with the laser from the critical areas, i.e., the regions with a particularly high risk of harboring residual tumor.

Prevention of Anterior Commissure Webs

a) In our experience, after resecting tumors of the anterior commissure and exposure of the thyroid cartilage, *regular swabbing of the fibrin in this area* will reduce the development of a web. After application of a topical anesthetic, a curved cotton wool applicator is introduced under endoscopic (90° telescope) control. This cotton wool can be soaked in a solution of gentamicin, cortisone, and alpha-chymotryptase. The cotton wool is firmly swept along the anterior commissure in order to remove fibrinous material and prevent adhesions that would result in synechiae (web) formation. This is the same procedure that is used to obtain a smear for cytology. The procedure is illustrated in Fig. 3.**25**.

We accept this essentially traumatic process because we believe the fibrin in the anterior commissure produces bridges which allow the overgrowth of epithelium, thus producing a web. The rationale is to delay the healing-over of epithelium in this area until the lateral edges of the commissure have started to heal. The treatment is repeated two to three times per week for 4–5 weeks. It is continued until wound healing and the filling of the wound defect with granulation tissue and subsequent epithelization starts. As soon as an epithelialized ridge of tissue as replacement for the vocal cord has formed, the topical treatment is stopped. Often only minor web formation occurs after this treatment, which is generally quite acceptable. The success of the treatment depends on the extent of the resection and on the individual wound-healing characteristics of the patient. The amount of care taken by the physician also plays an important role.

b) If a microlaryngoscopic assessment with biopsies is planned, the web prophylaxis, if at all necessary, is only started *after* this endoscopic control under general anesthesia. After operations through an external approach, a *silicone stent* can be sutured in the anterior commissure as prophylaxis for web formation. More recently we have employed this stenting technique also for transoral procedures with very promising results (Friedrich, 1996). In very extensive resections that go beyond the anterior glottic and subglottic area, a *Montgomery T-tube* can be used to prevent synechiae and stenoses. It should be left in situ for a period of 3–6 months.

Granulation tissue persisting for many months or an extensive web-like scar can on rare occasions lead to airway problems. Their removal with the laser serves to improve voice and airway and has the further advantage that residual tumor can be ruled out at the same time.

A close follow-up is required initially in 4-weekly intervals. This includes indirect or endoscopy (90° telescope) and smears for cytological examination. Additional, regular *Ultrasound examination* of the neck is necessary. Special emphasis is thereby put on the prelaryngeal soft tissues. For the early recognition of submucosal, extralaryngeal recurrent tumor growth CT or MRI are indicated in exceptional cases. Particularly in the first year of follow-up these imaging modalities, used in intervals of several months, have a place in the monitoring of the patient. One must, however, bear in mind that for technical reasons the obtained images are of limited value for the early detection of soft-tissue infiltration. We routinely use Ultrasound examinations of the cervical soft tissues and attach great value to the comparison of results obtained in serial studies during the course of the follow-up. Magnetic resonance imaging is only used in exceptional situations for the detection of submucosal soft-tissue recurrences (e.g. subglottic cancer).

Voice Rest or Voice Use?

In our opinion voice rest should only be recommended for patients with small, circumscribed mucosal defects that result from the removal of benign or superficially growing malignant lesions.

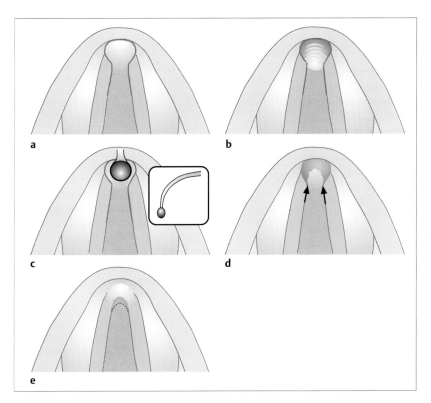

Fig. 3.25 Local aftercare to prevent web formation following the resection of a carcinoma of the anterior glottis and subglottis.
a There is a wound defect extending onto the inside of the thyroid cartilage after the resection of a carcinoma of the anterior glottis.
b Without local treatment, i.e., swabbing with a cotton wool applicator, a web would develop. The fibrin covering the wound would adhere to the contralateral side, granulation tissue would form abutting in the midline, and finally epithelium would grow over the granulations and result in solid tissue bridging the anterior glottis.

c A cotton wool applicator is introduced under endoscopic control. The fibrin is wiped off the anterior glottis close to the thyroid cartilage and adhesions are thereby prevented.
d In the meantime the epithelization progresses anteriorly in the area of the operated cords folds starting to cover the connective tissue that has already formed. The wound healing in the most anterior region in close proximity to the thyroid cartilage remains disturbed by the regular wiping with cotton wool swabs.
e After 4–5 weeks a web has developed. The extent of this scar formation depends on the individual healing characteristics of the patient and on the intensity of the postoperative local treatment.

In the case of larger wounds that are the consequence of more extensive tissue loss, patients are encouraged to make use of their voice. This will stimulate the formation of granulation tissue with subsequent transformation into hypertrophic connective tissue and finally a scar, which will eventually fill the defect and result in an improved vocal quality. The definitive result of the healing process cannot be predicted, due to the individually variable characteristics of healing and tissue regeneration. The individual response can range from the formation of hypertrophic granulation tissue to the complete absence of reparative processes.

If necessitated by tumor extent, a wide resection along the thyroid cartilage with sacrifice of the whole of true and false cord has become necessary, the desired formation of new tissue may not take place at all, due to the absence of a matrix. The end result in such cases is a mucosa-covered cartilaginous surface.

Severe dysphonia or even total aphonia can be the consequence. In these situations we prefer speech rehabilitation aiming at the acquisition of a supraglottic voice technique, similar to that of patients after extensive glottectomy. This may be in the form of the classic technique using the false cords, if these have been spared, or it can be achieved by acquiring the ability to approximate the petiole area of the epiglottis to the arytenoid cartilage(s) (see Chapter 5, p. 125 ff.).

T2 Glottic Tumors with Supraglottic and/or Subglottic Extent and Normal Cord Mobility

For all T2 carcinomas of the glottis primary laser surgery is advocated regardless of the pattern of tumor spread. It is of no significance whether it is a unilateral or bilateral tumor, whether it extends to involve supraglottis or subglottis, or whether it infiltrates anterior commissure or cricoid cartilage.

Operative Procedure

The surgical principles are the same as those that have so far been discussed in the context of other tumors. Superficially spreading carcinomas are ideally suited for laser surgery. Even if they cover vast areas of the endolarynx, they can be completely resected by performing a partial mucosectomy of the larynx (Fig. 3.**26**).

Superficial tumors which spread across the mucosa of the arytenoid cartilages far into the interarytenoid area can literally be peeled off. Arytenoid cartilages and their surrounding ligamentous and muscular structures, as well as their function can usually be preserved in the process of this dissection. Epithelization of the exposed cartilage is complete after 3–4 weeks.

As described above, the excision is performed in several individual pieces and the basal surfaces are stained with blue ink for better orientation by the pathologist. Exact topographical descriptions are very important on the pathology request form, but also in the patient's records, where the exact origin of the individual specimens must be noted in a schematic drawing of the larynx. The pathologist will be expected to comment on the grade of differentiation of the tumor, its depth of infiltration, and involvement of the basal resection margin. An examination of all the lateral margins does not make sense, as tumor is cut through on several occasions during the operation for such extensive lesions. In cases of doubt and in critical regions along the lateral resection line, the surgeon should excise additional specimens from the wound surface and submit them separately for histological examination.

Postoperatively, the surgeon must analyze the whole case by assimilating all the pieces of information that have been gathered before, during, and after surgery, almost in the form of a puzzle. The exact details of clinical and intraoperative findings that are recorded in the patient's file, in drawings, and on videotape are correlated with the histological findings and a precise and critical topographic comparison is made.

Our aims are thereby twofold. On the one hand, an assessment of localization and degree of the disease process within the larynx can be made. Similar to a map, this is plotted on a drawing of the larynx. On the other hand, certainty about the completeness of the resection along the basal surface can be obtained as far as at all possible. The larger the tumor and the more specimens we submit to the pathologist, the closer we get to the limits of histological processing and analysis. A small, well-circumscribed carcinoma of the glottis can easily be processed by routine serial sectioning in any pathological institute. If, however, five to ten specimens are submitted, the limits of what can be done are reached and the sections understandably become thicker. Biopsies should thus be limited to areas where the surgeon has doubts about the resection margin or critical regions in the wound for which objective proof of a complete resection is desirable. In view of the limitations of the histological assessment for these extensive tumors, one must remember the situation that would arise after a classical partial laryngectomy, provided this could still have been performed in the particular case. There the histological verification of a complete resection is also only possible with certain reservations. The therapeutic alternatives must also enter the equation. These are irradiation therapy with worse oncological results, and more commonly the total laryngectomy, which offers the greatest certainty for a complete resection of the cancer.

Additional resections. If the resection margin was not clear in one or more areas, further microlaryngoscopic resections can be carried out. The prerequisite for this is the meticulous labelling of the resected specimens. This may be supplemented by intraoperative video documentation, which can help to precisely locate the area from which an additional specimen has to be resected. Additional resections are rarely necessary after the resection of superficially growing tumors. This is also true for the microlaryngoscopic laser biopsies that are indicated if deeper infiltration was found in critical areas such as anterior commissure, arytenoid cartilages, or subglottis and the completeness of the resection could not be proved (Fig. 3.**27**). This is usually performed 4–6 weeks after the tumor resection.

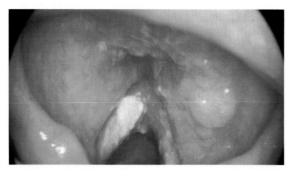
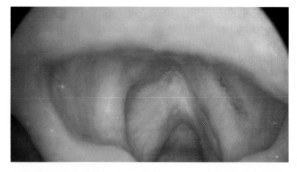

a   b

Fig. 3.**26** Superficially spreading carcinoma of glottis and supraglottis with bilateral extent (endoscopic view, 90° telescope). **a** Pretherapeutic findings of hyperplastic changes on the laryngeal surface of the epiglottis. The right side is more involved than the left. Lesions of leukoplakia are present on both vocal folds. The histology of these changes ranged from severe dysplasia to carcinoma in situ to infiltrating carcinoma. **b** The larynx after several microlaryngoscopic resections with the CO_2 laser in the area of supraglottis and glottis.

Carcinomas of the Glottis with Impaired Cord Movement ("T2b") and Fixed Vocal Cord (T3)

With regard to their superficial extension, these tumors are similar to the T2 lesions that have just been discussed. There is, however, definite clinical evidence of deeper infiltration in these cases. This can become manifest by
- markedly impaired cord movement or fixation of the vocal cord. This is usually easily diagnosed by laryngoscopic means;
- the results of radiographic investigations such as CT or MRI. It must, however, be remembered that false positive and false negative results are possible;
- intraoperative findings of direct tumor extent on the cut surface after a cut has been made through the lesion;
- postoperative histological examination of the specimen.

The variable extensions of glottic tumors along the mucosal surface and into underlying tissue can lead to an involvement of the following structures:
- musculature of the paraglottic space;
- perichondrium and/or thyroid cartilage can be reached, infiltrated, or broken through by tumor;
- arytenoid and/or cricoid cartilages can be involved or eroded;
- supraglottis and/or subglottis by superficial spread of tumor. Submucosal or intramuscular spread can also reach the paraglottic space in these regions;
- soft tissues of the neck via the cricothyroid membrane or after erosion of the thyroid cartilage.

These directions of potential tumor spread coincide with the most important subsites of the larynx, neighboring regions, and neighboring structures as included in the UICC/AJCC classification. Any tumor spread is carefully recorded in our oncology files, enabling the surgeon to exactly correlate clinical, intraoperative, and histological findings.

☞ In general any tumor of the larynx can be resected with oncological certainty from a purely surgical and technical point of view. The prerequisites are adequate exposure during the procedure and the absence of massive infiltration of the soft tissues of the neck (see Chapter 3, p. 37 ff.).

Operative Procedure (Fig. 3.27)

For T2 and T3 tumors of the glottis, incisions are made through the cancer to divide it into smaller portions. These are carried through laterally onto the thyroid cartilage and inferiorly onto the superior surface of the cricoid cartilage. The incision follows the extensions of the tumor and is made deeply into the musculature until a tissue layer is encountered which shows the reaction of normal tissue to the laser dissection under the microscope. If the musculature is invaded up to the perichondrium, the tumor is resected by dissecting along the inner table of the thyroid cartilage.

In the case of suspected infiltration of the thyroid cartilage or definite break-through, parts of the cartilage are included in the resection. An extra specimen resected from the neighboring prelaryngeal soft tissues can be used to verify the completeness of the resection.

Special Features of Resections in the Area of the Arytenoid Cartilages

It is important to realize that markedly impaired mobility of a vocal cord (T2b) or its fixation (T3) need not be the result of an infiltration of the arytenoid cartilage or of the cricoarytenoid joint. We follow our principle of individualized surgery which is adjusted to the extensions of the respective tumor. Thus, the resection of the arytenoid cartilage right at the beginning of the operation is avoided, unless the clinical situation clearly indicates that the preservation of the cartilage is no longer possible.

If the arytenoid cartilage, apart from its vocal process, is not per se involved in the disease process, an exploratory incision is made between the vocal process and the body of the arytenoid cartilage (Fig. 3.**28a**). During careful dissection under high magnification and with low laser power, it is usually quite easy to recognize the borders of the tumor and its extensions in a posterior direction toward the arytenoid cartilage and in a postero-inferior direction toward the cricoarytenoid joint. The arytenoid cartilage is, however, resected if it is found at surgery that the tumor has progressed submucosally into the direct vicinity of the arytenoid cartilage and thereby infiltrated its ligamentous and

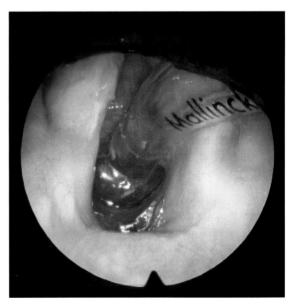
a

Fig. 3.**27** **a** Left vocal cord carcinoma with reduced mobility. The paraglottic space had been infiltrated; the tumor thickness was 14 mm. The individual steps of the operation are shown. **a** Microlaryngoscopy. The tube has been displaced anteriorly to expose the interarytenoid area and the posterior glottis.

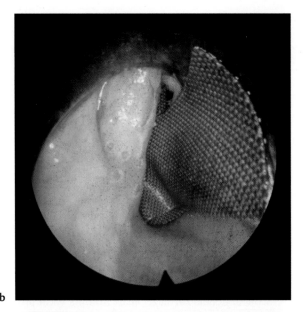

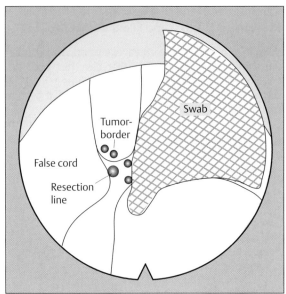

b

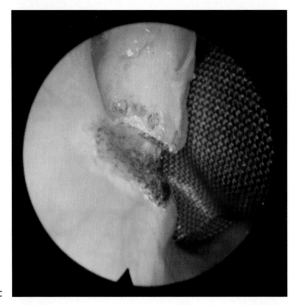

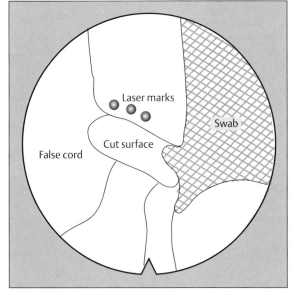

c

Fig. 3.**27** **b** Some marks are made with the laser to delineate the line of resection posteriorly and the macroscopically visible tumor borders anteriorly. **c** The incision is made anterior to the arytenoid cartilage through a healthy looking tissue layer.

The laser cut does not meet any resistance and is made with hardly any carbonization. This is evidence for a resection within normal tissue.

muscular attachments. The attempt should always be made to preserve the external, i.e., posterolateral mucosal surface of the arytenoid and to limit the resection to the parts of the cartilage that need to be removed from an oncological point of view. In the process it is not always necessary to completely expose the cricoid cartilage. By preserving the lateral mucosal cover of the arytenoid cartilage, the patient retains tissue that is functionally important for laryngeal protection during swallowing (Fig. 3.29). The temporary postoperative *lymph edema* contributes further to this effect.

⚡ The postoperative lymph edema can in some cases be so pronounced that the posterior laryngeal lumen becomes partially obstructed with resulting stridor. Usually the administration of intravenous steroids in a tapering dose is sufficient treatment. Laser excisions are only seldom necessary.

! During the resection of the arytenoid cartilage it is important to forcefully pull the cartilage in different directions with a grasping forceps in order to mobilize it. As the laser beam hits the tissue tangentially, this is the only way to cut "horizontally" through the cricoarytenoid joint under vision.

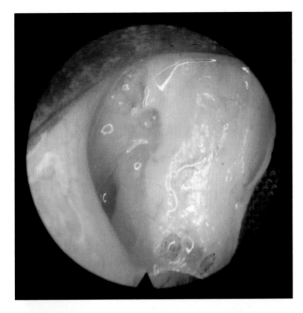

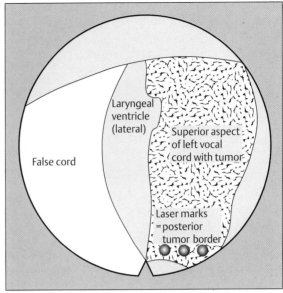

d

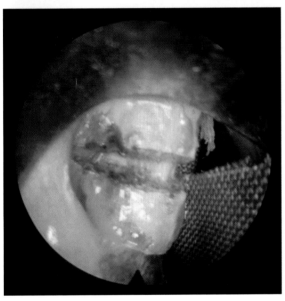

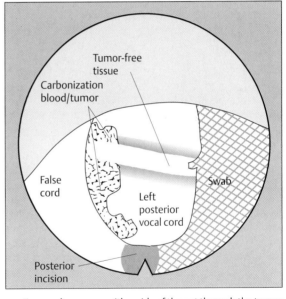

e

Fig. 3.**27**   **d** The lateral part of the superior surface of the vocal cord toward the laryngeal ventricle (sinus of Morgagni) is shown here. Massive submucosal tumor infiltration is found in this area. **e** Transection of the tumor approximately 6–7 mm anterior to the posterior line of resection. Signs of char formation can be seen on either side of the cut through the tumor. In the depth of the wound, however, healthy musculature becomes visible. The tumor extension into the paraglottic space is noticable.

The arytenoid cartilage must be mobilized in its entire circumference. Sometimes parts of the cartilage can be spared especially inferiorly. For this purpose a meticulous dissection under high magnification of the microscope is necessary. Occasionally, a curved pair of scissors can be useful in this operation.

As with all procedures, our aim is to preserve as much healthy tissue as possible. In the case of an arytenoidectomy, care must be taken not to cause too much damage with the tangential laser beam to the ligamentous and muscular structures surrounding the arytenoid cartilage. These are important for the histological examination. This dissection requires some experience if one wants to excise the arytenoid cartilage with simultaneous maximum preservation of tissue.

Resection of the Arytenoid Cartilage With Parts of the Subglottis and the Interarytenoid Area – Technical Details

1. The resection of the involved interarytenoid region is performed at the end of the operation. At that stage the endotracheal tube can be mobilized more liberally with the (small-caliber) laryngoscope than at

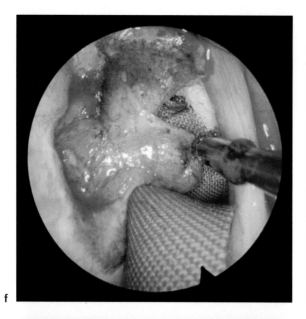

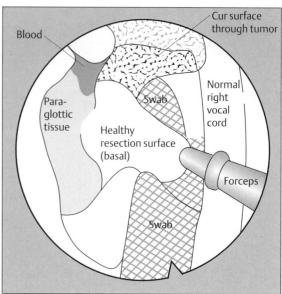

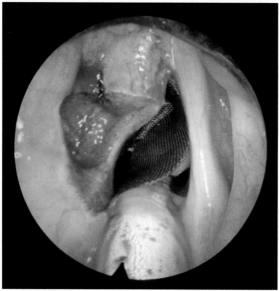

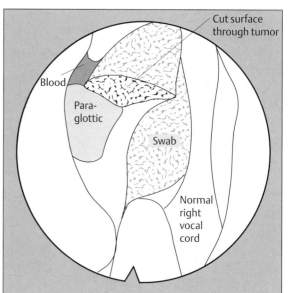

Fig. 3.**27**   **f** Resection of the dorsal part of the vocal cord with tumor. The specimen is retracted medially with the forceps. No tumor can be seen on the surface remaining after resection. This is the area which is of particular importance in the histological work-up. **g** The operative site after complete resection of posterior and middle segments of the vocal cord. Tumor-free muscle tissue remains on the lateral aspect in the depth of the wound (paraglottic space). Residual tumor can still be seen anteriorly.

the beginning of the procedure. It is gently pushed into the anterior and/or lateral wound cavity to gain access to the posterior glottis (Fig. 3.**28c**).

2. After the position of the tube has been adjusted, a medium-sized or small-caliber laryngoscope of extra length is introduced as far distally as possible and then lowered. This provides an improved exposure of the lateral and inferior aspects of the posterior larynx. Distending laryngoscopes are not as suitable for this area, as their distal opening is mostly oval-shaped. This means that the tips of the blades are too

wide to introduce them in a caudal direction in the area of the posterior larynx. One might think that the distending laryngoscope allows one to elevate the interarytenoid area with the posterior and at the same time to lift the endotracheal tube with the anterior blade. However, this is generally not possible in routine practice. The closed laryngoscope of extra length with a more round distal opening is better suited for this region (Fig. 1.**3b**).

3. Moist swabs must be carefully placed in the subglottic area in order to protect the cuff of the endotrache-

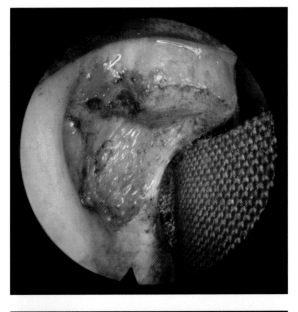
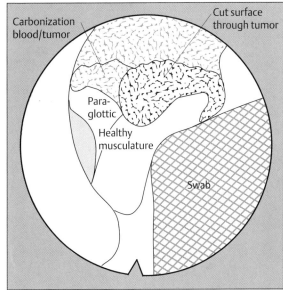
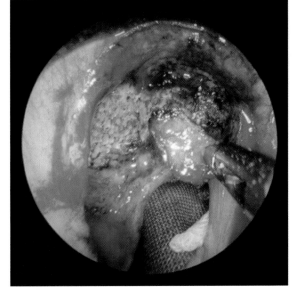
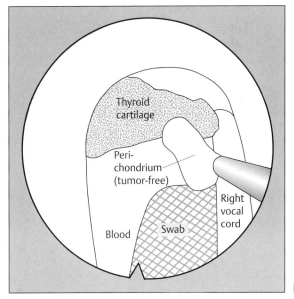

Fig. 3.**27**   **h** Detailed view of the left posterior area of resection in Fig. 3.27g. Tumor is visible in the lateral wound aspect with signs of carbonization. **i** The resection of the left anterior cord is performed close to the thyroid cartilage. Exposed cartilage and perichondrium on the left appear free of tumor. To the right the anterior specimen is retracted medially with a forceps. The basal resection margin appears clinically free of disease. This could be confirmed histologically.

al tube. On the one hand, this has the advantage of protection against the laser beam; on the other hand, it results in a better exposure of the operative field due to additional expansion of the lumen. This is particularly helpful for tumor extensions into the posterior subglottis. In some cases it may become necessary to improve the exposure by removing the endotracheal tube. The operation is then continued in the apneic phase and the patient later reintubated through the laryngoscope as described in a previous section.

4. By exerting pressure or traction on the surrounding healthy mucosa with the suction cannula or a grasping forceps, the tumor borders can often be better visualized.

Splitting of the interarytenoid bridge may become necessary if an adequate exposure through the small-caliber, extra-long laryngoscope cannot be achieved. This can occur in tumors with interarytenoid extensions that reach far inferiorly and occasionally involve the cricoid cartilage. The splitting is done very carefully and

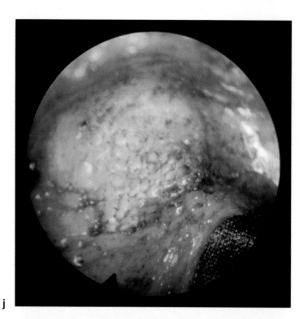

Fig. 3.**27** **j** Final situation after laser resection. The thyroid cartilage is widely exposed. Some muscular and ligamentous structures have been spared in the left subglottic area stretching anteriorly to below the anterior commissure. **k** Some fat can be seen prolapsing anteriorly in the area of the cricothyroid ligament. The lower border of the thyroid cartilage is clearly visible. The resection extended inferiorly onto the cricoid cartilage. Parts of the contralateral right cord have been removed as well. **l** Depth of infiltration of the six specimens.

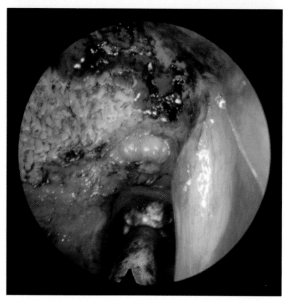

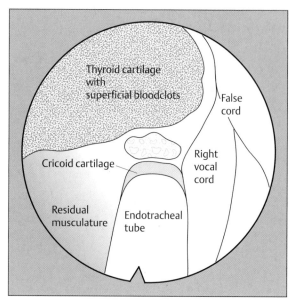

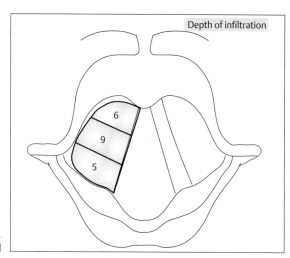

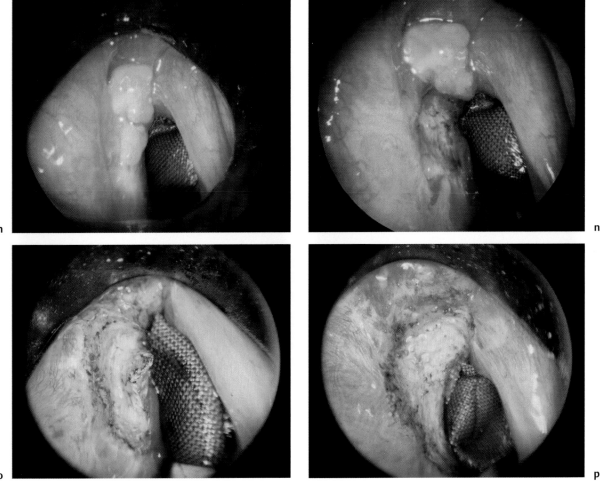

m

n

o

p

Fig. 3.**27** **m–p** Microlaryngoscopic resection of granulation tissue and postoperative assessment with laser biopsies (4–5 weeks after laser resection). m Granulation tissue can be seen anteriorly and in the middle of the area of the previous resection. n The partial resection of the granulations has been completed in the area of the former vocal fold. o Additional resection of approximately 2 mm of tissue from the floor of the wound (lateral) to definitely exclude a residual tumor. p The granulation tissue is also removed in the area of the anterior commissure together with a deeper layer of tissue. The thyroid cartilage is again exposed in the process. All specimens were free of tumor.

step by step similar to the division of the bar of tissue in a Zenker's diverticulum. It is only necessary to extend the incision so far as is required for a good exposure of the region of the cricoid cartilage through the newly positioned laryngoscope.

In exceptional cases the tumor spreads along the inner aspect of the interarytenoid area or along the cricoid cartilage toward the contralateral cricoarytenoid joint. Surgery in this area is challenging because of the risk of posterior glottic and subglottic stenosis.

More Technically Difficult, Critical Areas – Borderline Situations

Contralateral tumor spread or invasion of the supraglottis are no problems from a technical point of view.
- The involvement of the anterior commissure and subglottis have been discussed in detail in Chapter 3, p. 59.

- The invasion of the paraglottic space with breakthrough of tumor through the cricothyroid membrane into the soft tissues of the neck will be discussed, as will the extreme situation of subglottic and tracheal involvement.

Infiltration of the Paraglottic Space

The paraglottic space can be completely excised with the transoral technique of laser surgery. The dissection follows along the lamina of the thyroid cartilage up to its inferior edge.

The lower edge of the thyroid lamina may become eroded by tumor and the cancer can subsequently spread around the cartilage in an anterior and superior direction into the soft tissues of the neck.

Consequently, the inferior aspects of the thyroid cartilage should be resected until the surgeon comes upon tissue that is clearly tumor-free.

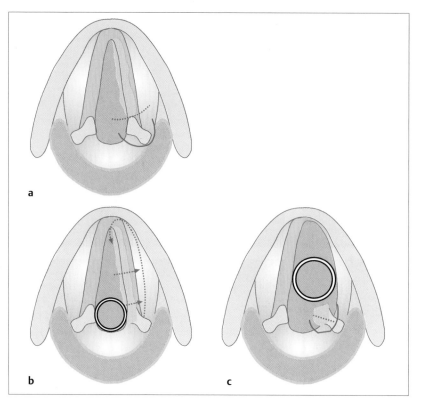

Fig. 3.**28** Extensive carcinoma of the right vocal fold with (queried) involvement of the arytenoid cartilage. **a** If the tumor reaches the area of the right arytenoid cartilage resulting in fixation or decreased movement, an initial exploratory incision is made immediately anterior to the body of the arytenoid. This uncovers the actual, submucosal, posterior extent of the tumor. Muscular and ligamentous structures in the proximity of the arytenoid can be infiltrated without actual involvement of the cartilage itself. It is often possible to preserve large parts or the entire arytenoid cartilage with this stepwise approach if the restriction of the movement was not caused by its immediate involvement in the disease process. **b** The anterior mass particularly of exophytic tumors is initially resected to improve the view in the case of extensive glottic lesions that spread to the arytenoid cartilages and the interarytenoid area. **c** The tube can then be displaced anteriorly in order to improve the exposure of the posterior larynx.

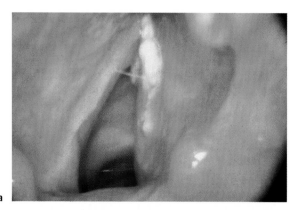
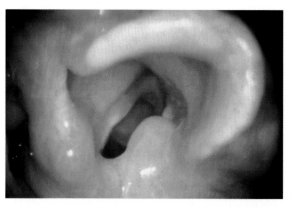

Fig. 3.**29** Carcinoma of the right vocal cord (T3) with fixed cord, before and after laser resection (Endoscopic view, 90° telescope). **a** Preoperative finding of a whitish tumor on the immobile right vocal cord. **b** The larynx after transoral microsurgical laser resection of vocal fold and parts of false cord and arytenoid cartilage on the right. Slight edema formation can be noticed in the area of the former arytenoid cartilage. In some patients this can be more extensive, depending on how much of the mucosa that covers the lateral aspect of the arytenoid cartilage could be preserved. The administration of cortisone is usually sufficient; only rarely are laser excisions of the edematous mucosa necessary. The left hemilarynx has been completely preserved anatomically and functionally. The patient received speech therapy and achieved a very satisfactory function of his voice. The voice training resulted in an approximation of the right arytenoid cartilage to the petiolus and thus the production of a "supraglottic voice" (see Fig. 5.**3**). Voice quality even after extensive transoral partial laryngectomies with the laser is comparable to that after conventional partial resections with reconstruction.

If the superior aspect of the cricoid cartilage is involved, tumor may have extended inferiorly along the external aspect of the cricoid. In these cases a partial resection of the cricoid cartilage must be performed.

Risks. More severe hemorrhages, especially arterial bleeding, can only be reached with great difficulty from the inside or not at all. Initial attempts to dissect out the bleeding vessel and ligate it with a clip are justifiable. Simultaneously applied external pressure can help in this dissection, for which the suction cannula and a peanut swab are very handy. Sometimes a small forceps is useful to spread the tissues in order to find the vessel. However, if these attempts fail, the lumen must be tamponaded, external pressure applied, and the *neck explored from the outside.*

Another indication for an external approach is the incomplete removal of tumor from the inside due to extensive growth into the soft tissues of the neck. In these cases the resection is continued and completed via a combined external, i.e., transcervical approach. It is usually sufficient to cover the resulting wound area from the inside with collagen mesh and fibrin glue. Additional cover from the outside in the form of a neck muscle sutured into the defect can be used as well. The external approach is routinely combined with a neck dissection. Due to the tumor break-through in the region of the cricothyroid membrane, the ipsilateral lobe of the thyroid gland is also included in the resection. A total laryngectomy should be avoided by all means, because the posterior larynx with the arytenoids can be preserved. Even a tracheotomy might not be necessary.

Extension Into Subglottis and Trachea

Technically difficult borderline situations for endoscopic surgery. Fortunately, tumor extensions far into the subglottis or even into the trachea are rare. They can be difficult to manage firstly because the exposure is often inadequate and secondly due to the cancer's potential for eroding the intercartilaginous membrane and breaking through into the paratracheal space. A resection as far down as the first and second tracheal ring is often possible when the extra-long, small-caliber laryngoscope is employed. If the endotracheal tube is in the way of the dissection, the operation can be continued in the apneic phase or during jet ventilation. Superficial tumors without deep infiltration can be dissected off the inside of the cricoid cartilage and the upper tracheal rings, even if they expand over a fairly large area. Good light and high magnification under the microscope are prerequisites for this surgery. Dissections in the area of the cricoid cartilage and proximal trachea are exceedingly difficult and require a lot of experience.

With this surgery it is especially important not to miss an infiltration of cartilage or break-through of tumor between cricoid cartilage and first tracheal ring.

Endoscopic inspection of the operative site through an intermittently introduced 25° telescope can be helpful in this operation.

For better exposure of the area between cricoid cartilage and posterior tracheal wall an endotracheal tube can be introduced into the esophagus and the cuff inflated at the level at which the resection takes place. As previously mentioned, this tumor rarely extends into the upper trachea. Primary tumors of the proximal trachea are even less common.

If the complete resection of the tumor is not possible due to poor exposure or tumor break-through into the paratracheal space, the neck must be opened from the outside. In a case like this, we first split the cricoid cartilage and the upper tracheal rings vertically in the midline and introduce a small endotracheal tube through the caudal part of this fissure. The tracheal walls are retracted with fine skin hooks and the operation is continued under the microscope with the laser. Depending on the extent of the resection, a primary closure or a tracheotomy as well as the creation of an epithelialized laryngotracheal fissure may become necessary. After a few months, this fissure can generally be closed without any problems, provided the patient has been tumor-free for some time. Even if relatively large parts of the cartilaginous rings have to be sacrificed due to infiltration by tumor, we do not immediately perform a laryngectomy. We approximate mucosa and skin of the neck in this situation and thus create an epthelialized fissure. Inferior to this an epithelialized stoma is created. The reconstructive procedure necessary to close the trachea in these cases is performed only after a tumor-free interval of 6–12 months.

Perioperative Measures After Extensive Transoral Partial Resections of the Larynx with Resection of One Arytenoid Cartilage for Advanced Glottic Carcinoma

Especially in elderly patients it is advisable to keep the patient intubated for 24 hours following an extensive partial resection of the larynx. If prolonged intubation is not an option, a tracheotomy should be considered. The conditions for early postoperative oral feeding are favorable if it was possible to preserve the epiglottis and a functional arytenoid cartilage during surgery. In spite of this we insert a nasogastric feeding tube in patients who have had a complete resection of an arytenoid cartilage.

Anterior glottic, subglottic, and lateral resections, even if they are extensive, have little impact on the function of the swallowing mechanism. However, problems arise from extensive resections in the posterior region of the larynx.

We only give *perioperative antibiotics* if large parts of the thyroid or cricoid cartilage have been exposed or resected. Even in extensive partial resections of the larynx it has never been necessary to externally ligate arterial feeding vessels for serious intraoperative hemorrhages or to do so prophylactically for the prevention of severe postoperative bleeding. There might, however, be a place for this approach in the surgery for tumors of the lateral pharyngeal wall that have infiltrated vastly into the soft tissues of the neck.

Postoperative Complications

Postoperative *hemorrhages* are very rare. They can usually be successfully managed by electrocautery at microlaryngoscopy. If at all, *edema* with a compromising effect on the airway is only seen after resection of the arytenoid cartilage with simultaneous preservation of the surrounding mucosa. It is usually caused by the interruption of lymph drainage. Normally, the administration of steroids is sufficient treatment and only seldom does the surgical removal of some of the edematous mucosa in the vicinity of the arytenoid cartilage become necessary.

It is difficult to predict the degree and duration of postoperative *aspiration*. There are patients who underwent a very extensive partial resection of the larynx (3/4 laryngectomy) and started swallowing successfully after 6–8 days. Others can present with swallowing problems for weeks after a simple hemilaryngectomy. Despite this we are of the opinion that the opportunity for a partial larynx resection should nevertheless be used as the primary method of treatment.

☞ For functional reasons a total laryngectomy should never be the next step but always the last. If subsequent to extensive resections radiotherapy is necessary for advanced neck disease, the insertion of a percutaneous endoscopic gastrostomy (PEG) feeding tube should be contemplated at an early stage of the treatment.

Late complications – laryngeal stenosis. The glottic and subglottic lumen is usually widened by the resection of the cancer. There is, however, a greater risk for fibrosis in the area between the arytenoid cartilages if more extensive resections are carried out in this area. The risk of stenosis also exists if the tumor necessitates an almost circumferential excision in the area of the cricoid cartilage. This risk is even higher in patients who have received previous irradiation to this area. We have operated on some patients with extensive recurrences after radiotherapy and with radiation-induced carcinomas (irradiation treatment 25 years previously). After multiple operations an almost complete endolaryngeal mucosectomy had been effected and additional resections of large parts of the soft tissues and the cartilage performed. Finally, a prolonged tumor-free period could be achieved, but one is then confronted with the problem of a secondary stenosis. Surprisingly, problems with aspiration occur less frequently in these cases.

☞ Fortunately, secondary stenosis is rare. It is found after extensive resection especially in the interarytenoid and subglottic areas. The formation of a stenosis is observed particularly after multiple procedures for recurrences in patients who received radiotherapy as primary treatment.

Supraglottic Carcinomas

Preoperative Diagnosis

Diagnostic procedures are largely determined by the eventual management strategy. This also applies to supraglottic carcinomas. If we see a chance for a partial resection of the larynx – this is usually the case – our routine diagnostic work-up consists of the following:

1. Tele-endoscopy with video documentation and smears for cytology. In the case of negative cytology another smear is taken and/or an intraoperative laser biopsy for frozen section obtained. Ultrasound examination of both sides of the neck are also routinely performed.

5. A panendoscopy is performed under general anesthesia before the transoral partial larynx resection with the laser.

Indications for imaging (MRI, CT). Tumor spread into the preepiglottic space, the paraglottic space, onto the anterior commissure, the arytenoid cartilage, or the thyroid cartilage are not contraindications for a curative resection with the laser via a transoral approach. Even for lesser degrees of infiltration of the soft tissue of the neck this technique can still be used in experienced hands. Thus, we do not routinely use imaging in the work-up of these patients. Radiographic investigations, however, play a role when massive tumor infiltration into the neck is suspected. In this situation the limits for a curative partial resection exclusively via a transoral route are reached. Preoperative information on the exact tumor extent helps to improve the surgical planning with routes of approach from inside and outside.

☞ The basic rule is still for the surgeon to be guided by the intraoperative findings. As previously described, this entails following the tumor and adjusting the operation to the respective extensions of the cancer.

Supraglottic Carcinomas (T1, Carcinoma In Situ)

Operative Procedure

Small, well-circumscribed tumors of the supraglottis are rather rare. They can be resected in one piece, similar to a lesion on the vocal cord (Fig. 3.**30**).

Suprahyoid Epiglottis and False Cord Area

The resection can technically be easily performed. The advantage of this region is the fact that wide margins can be kept without having to worry about functional implications, as in the case of glottic lesions. The histological documentation of a complete resection with clear margins can be made safely and with ease (Fig. 3.**31**).

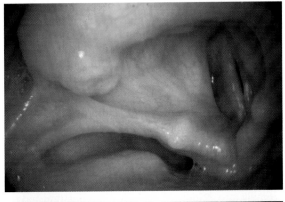

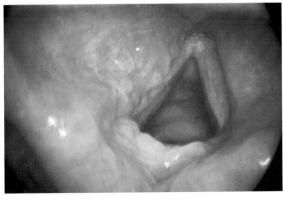

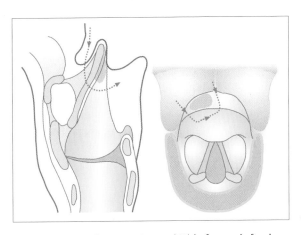

Fig. 3.**30** Supraglottic carcinoma (T1) before and after laser resection. **a** The preoperative photographic documentation through the 90° telescope shows a circumscribed polypoid tumor of the left suprahyoid epiglottis. **b** This shows the findings after transoral partial laser resection of the epiglottis. **c** A circumscribed tumor of the suprahyoid epiglottis can be safely and completely resected in one piece along the resection line shown in the drawing.

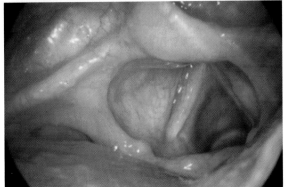

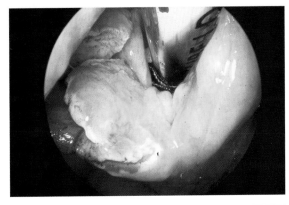

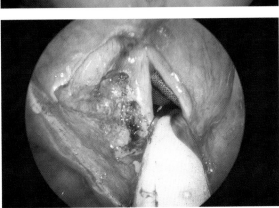

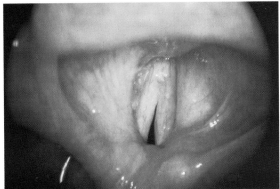

Fig. 3.**31** Supraglottic carcinoma left, pT1. **a** Preoperative endoscopic view (90° telescope) of the ventricular band carcinoma. **b** The intraoperative view shows a step of the block-wise resection of the tumor posteriorly. **c** Aspect of the wound cavity after laser surgical removal in several pieces. **d** Postoperative endoscopic view (90° telescope) of the definite healing with a very satisfactory functional glottis.

Infrahyoid Epiglottis

Deep infiltration of tumor in the area around the petiole is difficult to assess preoperatively. Considerable problems can arise when the distinction between a T1 tumor and a T3 lesion (infiltration of the preepiglottic space) has to be made.

Early stages of carcinoma and slightly more extensive but superficial disease can in principle be excised with preservation of the suprahyoid epiglottis. However, infiltration of the preepiglottic space must always be expected from tumors in the area of the petiole (Fig. 3.**32**).

The dissection of a carcinoma of the petiole with preservation of the suprahyoid epiglottis can be rendered difficult by suboptimal exposure. The tumor can usually be visualized on the mucosal surface either through a closed or a distending laryngoscope. However, the dissection of the deeper-lying tissues can be difficult or even impossible due to inadequate exposure and thus lack of oncological safety. The almost impossible angle makes surgical access difficult, despite external pressure on the laryngeal skeleton.

We first attempt to expose the area around the petiole and make an incision into the mucosa around the tumor in order to establish whether the view of the operative field is adequate (Fig. 3.**33**). If it is not a superficial carcinoma, but a deeply infiltrating process and the exposure is not sufficient, the access route can immediately be changed to an approach from above through the vallecula. This access route is depicted in Fig. 3.**34**. It is simpler and safer even in cases of difficult exposure of the endolarynx and particularly the anterior commissure.

Procedure in detail. The vallecula is entered. The suprahyoid epiglottis is split sagittally and after conventional electrocautery to the vascular pharyngoepiglottic folds and the medial glossoepiglottic fold, these are transsected. The distending laryngoscope is subsequently advanced (Fig. 3.**37c**). One can now clearly see the cut surface through the epiglottic cartilage, the preepiglottic fat, and the laryngeal surface of the infrahyoid epiglottis with the tumor. Further steps are the same as in Fig. 3.**34**. The tumor is cut through in a sagittal plane. The dissection proceeds in an inferior direction. Depending on the extent of the tumor, horizontal cuts are indicated through the bulk of the lesion.

Bigger tumors with an infiltrative growth pattern can erode through the epiglottic cartilage and fill the preepiglottic space almost completely. This extent can be clearly recognized intraoperatively. The excision is made oncologically safe with a margin of 5–10 mm. No functional impairments are to be expected from this operation.

Microinvasion of the preepiglottic space can only be diagnosed histologically. For this reason, 5–10 mm of the preepiglottic space are usually included in the resection even if the epiglottic cartilage appears intact at operation. That way invasion which is only detect-

able histologically is safely recognized. The dissection is continued anteroinferiorly onto the thyroid cartilage at the level of the anterior commissure. An oncologically safe resection of the tumor is thereby effected anteriorly at the level of the false cords and inferiorly at the upper level of the anterior commissure.

Perioperative and postoperative measures and aftercare. Neither a prolonged intubation over 24 hours, or a tracheotomy is necessary after partial resections of the epiglottis or the false cords. Antibiotic prophylaxis and nasogastric feeding tube are also not generally indicated. The patient can usually be discharged after a few days in hospital. Secondary hemorrhages are extremely rare. After the histological examination and the analysis of all the information on the case by the surgeon, a plan for the aftercare is devised. The management is the same as for glottic carcinomas. The functional rehabilitation of the patient is usually completed after a relatively short period.

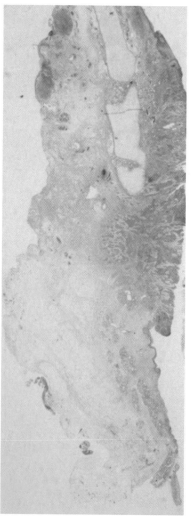

Fig. 3.**32** Sagittal section through the epiglottis (after Goldner): squamous cell carcinoma with infiltration of the preepiglottic space. The charred surface along the line of resection in the preepiglottic space is free of tumor.

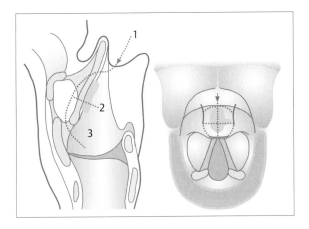

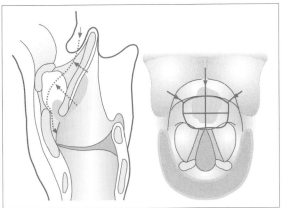

Fig. 3.**33** Supraglottic carcinoma (T1, area of petiole). The attempt is made to resect the tumor and parts of the preepiglottic space with preservation of the suprahyoid epiglottis. The anterior false cords are partially included in the resection. The prerequisite for this is the adequate exposure of the tumor in the petiole area through a distending or a tubular laryngoscope. This must provide unimpaired access, so that the resection of the cancer even within the preepiglottic space becomes possible. The resection is simply extended anteriorly if break-through into the preepiglottic space has occurred. The operation starts with an incision superiorly through healthy tissue (1). A transection of the tumor follows (2). This allows the assessment of the depth of extension toward the preepiglottic space. Intraoperatively the resection is adjusted according to the extent of tumor infiltration that is seen under the high magnification of the operating microscope. The inferior resection completes the operation (3).

Fig. 3.**34** Supraglottic carcinoma with infiltration of the preepiglottic space (T3). Especially in cases of unequivocal clinical or radiological evidence of massive infiltration of the preepiglottic space, the entire epiglottis is resected. The first incision is made in the vallecula (1). Perpendicular to this a cut is made through the middle of the epiglottis (2). The suprahyoid segments of the epiglottis are now removed bilaterally. The resection proceeds caudally in a stepwise fashion. Vertical and horizontal cuts (3) are laid through the tissue and the tissue blocks removed. The operation may extend onto the hyoid bone anteriorly. This can be partially resected if an infiltration by tumor is suspected. Inferiorly the resection follows the inside of the thyroid cartilage toward the anterior commissure (4). If there is a suspicion of superficial or submucosal spread to the anterior glottis, this region is included in the resection. Even the extensive tumor involvement of the glottis is not a contraindication for a partial laser resection.

Supraglottic Carcinomas

(T2–T4, Fig. 3.35–3.40)

For T2 supraglottic cancers and T3 lesions (based on the infiltration of the preepiglottic space) with normal mobility of both arytenoid cartilages, the diagnostic and surgical management is identical to that of T1 tumors of the supraglottis. The extent of the transoral endoscopic resection is that of the classic supraglottic laryngectomy after Alonso, except for the preservation of the tumor-free thyroid cartilage.

Problems of aspiration must be expected during the first few days after this extensive resection, which includes epiglottectomy with or without false cord and aryepiglottic fold. We usually insert a feeding tube and keep it in for a few days postoperatively, although this is not necessary in younger patients despite complete resection of the epiglottis. A tracheotomy is (usually) not required.

Operative Technique

The surgical procedure is the same as the technique described for advanced glottic carcinomas (T3 and T4). The operation proceeds from cranial to caudal and the resection should be limited to one level at a time (Fig. 3.**34**, 3.**36**, and 3.**37c**). The laryngoscope can be advanced subsequent to the resection of one level and the deeper-lying regions resected in a similar fashion.

If thyroid or arytenoid cartilages are infiltrated by tumor, they are included in the resection. During the resection of parts of the thyroid cartilage, one must beware of extralaryngeal vessels. If tumor has broken through the thyrohyoid membrane, it is followed as far into the neck as possible. The resection can reach all the way into the subcutaneous tissue of the neck skin.

In the case of a large, exophytic tumor it may be necessary to debulk the cancer by horizontal and vertical incisions through the tumor mass. The exact borders of the tumor can then be recognized with greater certainty and ease (Fig. 3.**5**).

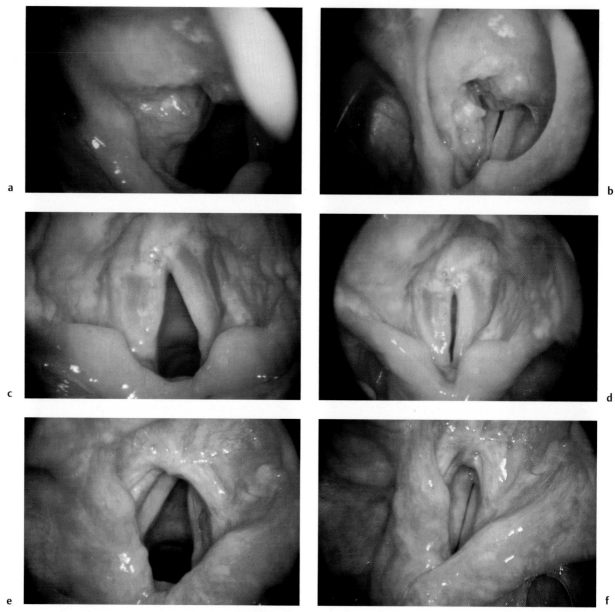

Fig. 3.**35** Preoperative and postoperative documentation of a supraglottic carcinoma (T3). **a** and **b** Preoperative endoscopic (90° telescope) findings of an exophytic cancer of the infrahyoid epiglottis on both sides. The lesion involves the left false cord, the paraglottic space, and reaches onto the arytenoid cartilage. **c** and **d** Two weeks after laser resection an tele-endoscopic view is obtained in inspiration and phonation.

Fibrin covering the wound can be seen bilaterally. **e** and **f** Endoscopic view 24 months after the operation in inspiration and phonation. A ridge of scar tissue has formed in the area of the former epiglottis. Both vocal folds move normally and a complete closure of the cords is possible. No functional impairment resulted.

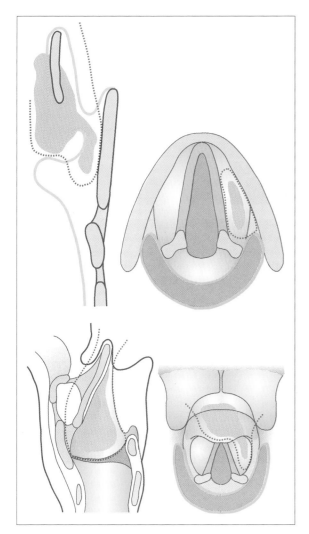

Fig. 3.**36** Extensive supraglottic carcinoma with infiltration of the preepiglottic and the right paraglottic space. The different views show the tumor extent and the resection line that was adjusted to the extensions in the respective directions. Large parts of the preepiglottic space, of anterior glottis, and of the right paraglottic space have to be sacrificed in this operation. As previously described, the resection is performed in several tissue blocks and proceeds level by level in a cranio-caudal direction. The position of the laryngoscope must be adjusted several times in the course of the operation. Corresponding to the progression of the resection the laryngoscope is advanced deeper and deeper. In order to resect the paraglottic space it needs to be inserted from an oblique angle from the corner of the mouth.

Fig. 3.**37** Supraglottic carcinoma (T3) with bilateral extensions. The main origin is from the right side; the right paraglottic space and the preepiglottic space are infiltrated. Preoperative, intraoperative, and postoperative endoscopic views (90° telescope) are shown. **a** Preoperative photo taken in inspiration. **b** During phonation the tumor on the right laryngeal surface of the epiglottis becomes visible. It had a partly ulcerating, partly exophytic, and partly deeply infiltrating growth pattern. The cancer extended onto the left epiglottis, the medial aspect of the right aryepiglottic cord, and the right false cord. Inferiorly the tumor had grown lateral to the vocal cord into the paraglottic space more so on the right than the left. **c** Intraoperative findings. After resection of the superior part of the epiglottis (suprahyoid), the tumor (in the infrahyoid epiglottis), the epiglottic cartilage, and the wide front of infiltration into the preepiglottic space become visible. **d** The situation at the end of the operation. The thyroid cartilage has been exposed and the vocal cord have been largely preserved. The wound is an extensive cavity combining supraglottis and paraglottic space. **e** Findings during inspiration, a few weeks after the transoral laser resection. Both arytenoid cartilages have been preserved. **f** A complete glottic closure is achieved during phonation. Fibrinous membranes are still noticable in the area of resection. g and h Six weeks after laser resection in inspiration (**g**) and phonation (**h**). The residual larynx is completely healed. A ridge of scar tissue has formed in the region of the right vocal cord. The functional postoperative results were highly satisfactory.   ▶

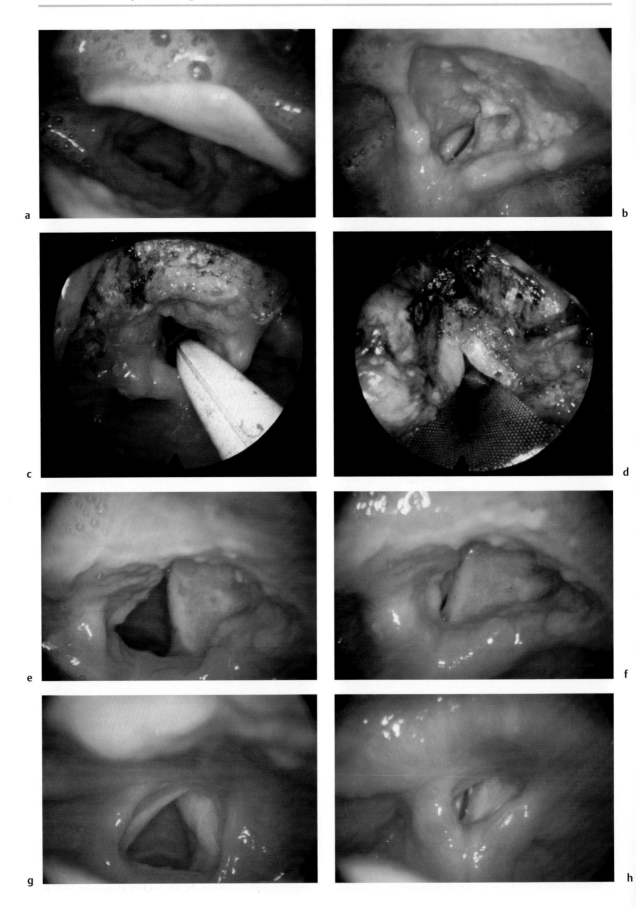

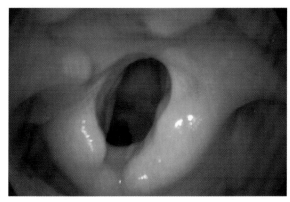

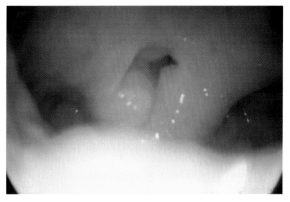

Fig. 3.**38** View of a larynx after laser resection of an extensive bilateral supraglottic and glottic carcinoma. In this patient the only laryngeal structures that could be spared were both arytenoid cartilages. An almost complete protective closure of the glottic aperture can be seen during phonation. **a** In inspiration. **b** In phonation.

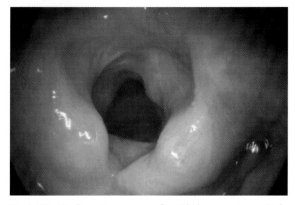

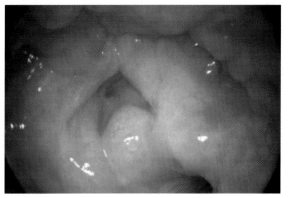

Fig. 3.**39** Findings in a patient after 3/4 laryngectomy. Only the right arytenoid cartilage with a small part of the right vocal cord could be preserved in this case. Mucosal edema can be seen on the left in the area of the arytenoid cartilage, which was completely removed. Complete glottic closure is, nevertheless, achieved by the right arytenoid cartilage. The patient does not experience any impairment of respiration or swallowing. After speech therapy, he regained an easily intelligible voice, which allowed him to continue his work. **a** Endoscopic view during inspiration. **b** During phonation.

If intraoperative bleeding occurs from the superior laryngeal artery, we control it with a vascular clip. In the case of a resection with inclusion of the soft tissues of the neck, during which larger vessels were coagulated, it is recommended to apply collagen mesh and fibrin glue to the wound surface.

Advantages of Transoral Supraglottic Partial Laryngectomy Over the Classic Supraglottic Laryngectomy After Alonso

The transoral approach usually allows the surgeon to preserve the thyroid cartilage, the superior laryngeal artery and vein, and the superior laryngeal nerve. The view through the microscope and the almost bloodless dissection enable the surgeon to limit the resection to those structures of the larynx that are affected by the tumor. This implies a high degree of oncological certainty and maximum preservation of function. There is no tendency to overtreat the patient with this approach. Other advantages are the minimal blood loss, no tracheotomy, better and faster rehabilitation of swallowing, shorter operating time, hospital stay, and illness, lower incidence of secondary stenoses, and a better functioning voice.

Extension of tumor to neighboring structures such as oropharynx or hypopharynx, infiltration or break-through of the thyroid cartilage, tumor breaking through thyrohyoid membrane or cricothyroid membrane, infiltration of the paraglottic space, and fixation of an arytenoid cartilage are all not contraindications for us to perform a transoral laser-surgical partial resection of the larynx (Fig. 3.**35**–3.**41**).

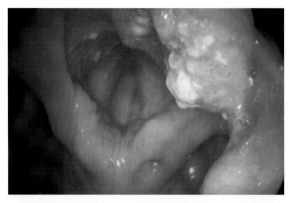

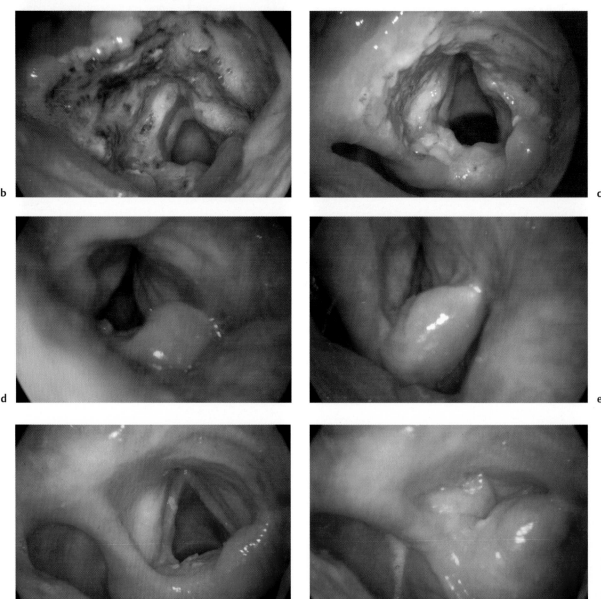

Fig. 3.**40**   Double pathology of the supraglottis (carcinoma of the right epiglottis and the area of the left arytenoid cartilage) The patient received a transoral laser resection, bilateral functional neck dissections, and postoperative irradiation. **a** Preoperative finding (endoscopic view, 90° telescope). **b** One week after laser resection: fibrin is covering the wound and the thyroid cartilage is exposed. **c** During the radiotherapy, which was necessary because of bilateral cervical metastases, a mucositis with layers of fibrin is noticable. **d** and **e** Three months after completion of radiotherapy. Edema can still be seen at endoscopy in inspiration and phonation. **f** and **g** The endoscopic aspect after 1 year is identical to the one after 15 years. Some mucus can be seen on the left cord and in the posterior commissure (**f**).

Conventional supraglottic partial resections in the form of a 3/4 or 4/5 laryngectomy are only rarely performed in patients with such extensive tumors, and traditionally a total laryngectomy is the treatment of choice in these cases.

Limitations of Transoral Lasersurgery for Extensive Supraglottic Tumors

The primary obstacle is, in analogy to all the other sites, the unfavorable exposure. Although with adequate experience, larger tumors can be resected through a small-caliber laryngoscope, this is not recommended for surgeons with limited experience. An operation from an external approach is advisable in this situation also with the aim of partial organ preservation.

Further limitations for this method arise from massive infiltration of the large vessels in the neck. This always requires a combined approach from the inside and the outside.

An extreme situation from a functional aspect arises from the massive infiltration of the tongue base by an extensive supraglottic tumor and simultaneous fixation of the arytenoid cartilage. This requires large parts of the base of the tongue and the arytenoid cartilage to be included in the resection. The consequence is a relatively high risk of aspiration.

Examples of borderline indications and contraindications are shown in Fig. 3.**41** and 3.**42**.

Perioperative and Postoperative Measures After Extended Supraglottic Partial Resections of the Larynx (3/4 and 4/5 Laryngectomy)

The extended supraglottic laser resection must be seen as a last alternative to a total laryngectomy. The measures taken during postoperative treatment are the same as for the resection of T2 and T3 supraglottic tumors, unless large parts of the tongue base or an arytenoid cartilage have been resected in the course of the operation. Longer lasting swallowing problems must be expected if very extensive resections have been performed which reached far into the oropharynx (infiltration of base of tongue) or into the hypopharynx. This problem becomes particularly severe if an arytenoid cartilage has been removed in addition. Several factors determine how long the feeding tube should be kept in situ, whether there is an indication for a PEG, or whether a temporary tracheotomy is necessary. These are:
- Age of the patient,
- Pulmonary reserve and lung function,
- Necessity for postoperative irradiation, for example, for advanced disease in the neck,
- Degree of intraoperative hemorrhages,
- Presence of a bleeding tendency or coagulopathy (patients on Warfarin or hemodialysis), etc.

All these criteria need to be weighed carefully before the decision is made to subject the patient to a PEG or a tracheotomy. In any case, a prolonged intubation of 24 hours should be envisaged after such extensive surgery, especially in elderly patients. A longer stay of these patients in the intensive care ward is usually necessitated by concurrent medical problems rather than related to the surgery. Once these patients are back in the normal ward, they require close observation because of the risk of secondary hemorrhages, aspiration, etc. Antibiotics are given for a period of approximately 1 week.

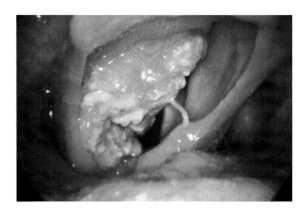

Fig. 3.**41** Extensive laryngeal carcinoma with spread across the midline in the area of the supraglottis (Endoscopic view, 90° telescope). On the left the tumor involved the entire supraglottis, glottis, and arytenoid area. It extended into the interarytenoid region. This is an example of a tumor where a partial resection of the larynx is still possible with sparing of the right arytenoid cartilage and parts of true and false cord as well as aryepiglottic fold on the same side.

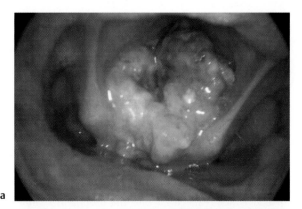

a

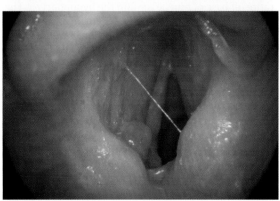

b

Fig. 3.**42** **a** Laryngeal carcinoma with airway obstruction in an 80-year-old patient. Almost the entire larynx, particularly the posterior part, is obstructed (Endoscopic view, 90° telescope). Although a complete curative resection of the tumor is technically possible, the patient would suffer from severe aspiration postoperatively, as large parts of both arytenoid cartilages would have to be removed. In this case the tumor was debulked liberally to spare the patient a tracheotomy. Subsequent irradiation treatment could be given due to a good general condition of the patient. This resulted in a tumor-free period of 1 year. **b** Left posteriorly a tumor recurrence can be noted after 1 year. This was removed with the laser. The patient survived for almost 3 years and died of an unrelated cause.

Postoperative Complications

- Surgical emphysema is rather rare. It is treated expectantly and does not require any active intervention.
- Secondary hemorrhages occur from predeliction sites, namely anterolateral to the area of the arytenoid cartilage and superior and lateral to the upper edge of the thyroid cartilage. The problem is managed at microlaryngoscopy. The source of bleeding is located and the vessel diathermized or clipped. Finding the vessel may be difficult due to the relative hypotension during general anesthetic.
- Severe aspiration can lead to the development of aspiration pneumonia or atelectases. However, this occurs rather infrequently. The management consists of tracheotomy and conservative therapy with antibiotics, inhalations, physiotherapy, etc.
- Dyspnea is extremely rare in these patients. It occurs in cases of extensive edema of both arytenoid cartilages. Treatment measures should be stepwise in the following order: administration of steroids (often successful on its own), bilateral laser excision of edematous mucosa in the area of the arytenoid cartilages (rarely necessary), tracheotomy (extremely rarely necessary).

Postoperatively, patients complain surprisingly little of pain but commonly of excessive secretions. This is even more so in patients who had a resection of an oropharyngeal or hypopharyngeal carcinoma. This is not a phenomenon of secretions from the wound surface, but more the result of the patients' difficulty with the swallowing of their own saliva. On the one hand, this may be caused by the fear of aspiration. Severe bouts of cough due to aspiration are very unpleasant for the postoperative patient. On the other hand, the swallowing of saliva may cause pain and is therefore avoided. In extreme situations the mucus that collects in the pharynx can inspissate and form a mucous plug, which can result in airway obstruction.

Humidification of the inspired air is therefore very important. The patients are encouraged to start swallowing their saliva at an early stage after surgery, despite the unpleasant side effects. For cases of excessive secretions, i.e., production of saliva we give anticholinergic drugs such as scopolamine.

Transoral Laser Microsurgery for Hypopharyngeal Carcinomas

Preoperative (Intraoperative) Diagnosis

If a squamous cell carcinoma of the hypopharynx is suspected, the following investigations should be performed:
- Endoscopy (90° telescope) of larynx and pharynx
- Photo and/or video documentation

✍ Endoscopy on the awake patient has certain advantages. During phonation the pyriform sinus and the postcricoid region open up and allow better assessment of the inferior extent of the tumor. At the same time the mobility of the arytenoid cartilages can be evaluated. In general a better overview is obtained at endoscopy in the awake patient compared to direct inspection of the hypopharynx under general anesthesia, where often only part of the whole disease process can be seen at a time.

- Smears for cytology from the hypopharynx can often be taken without application of a topical anesthetic. If the results from cytology are negative, the smear is repeated or a biopsy for histology is obtained under local or general anesthesia. The patient is usually admitted to hospital for the latter. An incisional biopsy with the laser can also be obtained at the time of curative resection and sent for frozen-section examination.

The extent of any further pretherapeutic diagnostic investigations depends mainly on the type of the subsequent therapy being envisaged.

Indications for Partial Pharyngolaryngeal Resection

The pretherapeutic assessment comprises an endoscopic examination under general anesthesia and the use of CT-imaging. The results of these investigations determine whether a partial resection is still possible and justifiable. Diagnostic errors can arise due to the special growth characteristics of the tumors in the hypopharynx and due to the limitations of the preoperative investigations despite the use of highly advanced technologies.

Several authors (Glanz 1999; Zbären, Egger 1997) have demonstrated in histological studies that hypopharyngeal tumors have certain characteristics that distinguish them from other sites in the upper aerodigestive tract. At an early stage these tumors show signs of infiltrative growth and a strong tendency for *submucosal spread*. These characteristics must be respected in the decision on the feasibility of a partial resection. The tumor extension on the mucosal surface, as seen by the examiner, is only seldom a reflection of the true tumor extent. Carcinomas of the pyriform sinus can invade the paraglottic and preepiglottic space, the area of the arytenoid cartilages, the thyroid cartilage, or the soft tissues of the neck without any evidence on endoscopy. Only if there is extensive infiltration of, for example, the cricoarytenoid joint, will the deep invasion of the tumor become clinically apparent by impaired mobility or fixation of the arytenoid cartilage. Most laryngologists would agree that such tumor extent goes beyond the limits of a partial pharyngolaryngeal resection.

Imaging techniques such as CT and MRI are required for more precise evaluation of the tumor extension during the pretherapeutic work-up. The areas of greatest concern are tumor spread in an inferior direction, contralateral spread, extralaryngeal extensions, and infiltration of the thyroid cartilage. Impressive images have recently demonstrated the progress that has been made with CT and MRI. Studies comparing the imaging results with the histological findings on the surgical specimen confirm the value and limitations of imaging for the pretherapeutic staging.

✍ The authors of several studies have demonstrated that both overestimation and underestimation of true tumor extension can occur. False positive results were found in the presence of edema and inflammatory changes surrounding the tumor. False negative findings occurred in cases of small tumor foci, submucosal spread or cartilage invasion.

If the tumor proves larger than expected during attempted partial pharyngolaryngeal resection, a conventional radical procedure or a radiochemotherapy can still be performed.

⚡ The more serious diagnostic dilemma is the overestimation of the tumor extent during the pretherapeutic staging. This can potentially lead to the unnecessary removal of an organ.

✍ If the tumor involves the lateral wall of the pyriform sinus and there is suspicion of deep infiltration, CT or preferably MRI should be performed to identify tumor break-through into the soft tissues of the neck (Fig. 3.1b). This knowledge is of great importance for the surgical planning of a transoral laser procedure.

If surgery is still indicated, a combined approach should be chosen for these rare cases. (See above). A neck dissection is always performed at the same time in these cases.

Ultrasound examination in the B-scan mode is the method of choice for us for the assessment of cervical metastases. This is especially useful for the detection of clinically occult metastases (N0). A diagnostic-therapeutic endoscopy is planned if a partial resection of hypopharynx and larynx seems feasible. This is usually performed after the initial suspicion of a malignancy has been confirmed by cytological or histological proof of squamous cell carcinoma. The aim of this procedure is the full assessment of the extent of the tumor and, if circumstances allow, its treatment by complete, curative resection during the same general anesthetic.

Endoscopy of Upper Digestive Tract and Entire Respiratory Tract (Microlaryngoscopy, Oro- and Hypopharyngoscopy, Esophagoscopy, and Bronchoscopy)

Aims

- If previous cytological smears or biopsies taken endoscopically under topical anesthetic have been negative, an *incisional* biopsy by laser is obtained at microlaryngoscopy for frozen-section examination.
  - If it is a circumscribed lesion, an *excisional* biopsy is done with the laser.
  - If extensive disease is encountered, an incisional biopsy is performed by laser.
- The tumor extent is assessed, for example, in case of a carcinoma of the pyriform sinus, the larynx, postcricoid area, and esophagus must be evaluated for possible invasion by tumor.

The question to be answered is whether or not the lesion can be resected with preservation of function.

☝ At the beginning of the operation the laryngopharyngoscope should always be inserted into the uninvolved hypopharynx. This reduces the chance of traumatizing tumor tissue and thus reduces subsequent bleeding. The inferior extent of the tumor, toward the esophageal inlet, can hence be assessed with greater accuracy.

- A second primary must be excluded. If a second primary is clinically suspected or proved by frozen section, this has certain consequences for the patient. These are discussed in more detail in Chapter 3, p. 37f.

Operative Preparations

- Aspects of the preferred anesthesia are discussed in more detail in Chapter 4 (p. 116ff). General anesthetic with endotracheal intubation (MLT tube) is commonly used.
- The instrumentation is detailed in Chapter 1, p. 3ff. The use of the distending laryngopharyngoscope (Fig. 1.**4a**) is preferable. Only if the transoral exposure is difficult is a medium- or small-caliber closed laryngoscope used. A disadvantage is the impaired general exposure, which makes the procedure more difficult. The same microinstruments are used as for laryngeal surgery.
- Findings and surgical procedure should be demonstrated and documented on video.

Laser Surgical Procedure

The laser is used either in continuous mode or in superpulse for this dissection. The power setting is adjusted to the tissue that is to be transected. For the dissection through healthy tissue low power is adequate, whereas higher power is required for cutting through tumor tissue.

Dissection Technique

It is generally recommended to resect step by step in a cranio–caudal direction. The tumor is removed "blockwise" and layer by layer. For instance, the resection of a pyriform sinus carcinoma starts laterally and then follows the anterior tumor extent ending medially (Fig. 3.**43b**). At the beginning a maximum thickness of approximately 1 cm is resected at a time for each layer. The resection progresses layer by layer from proximal to distal. One must avoid dissecting too deeply (caudally) at any one particular point, where the exposure becomes limited and extensive bleeding may occur.

The dissection may only proceed inferiorly as far as good exposure and accessibility of the tissues in the dissection plane can be guaranteed. In the process the tumor is divided in a mosaic-like fashion by horizontal and vertical cuts. The border between tumor and healthy tissue can be well identified on the tissue section. The distending laryngopharyngoscope should generally be positioned so that a margin of normal tissue of approximately 10 mm remains between the blade of the speculum and the edge of the visible tumor. The incision into the mucosa must be made under the *highest possible magnification* of the microscope.

Advantages:
- Appearances of early pathological changes of the mucosa in the proximity of the tumor must be looked for carefully under maximum magnification.

☝ These lesions commonly form recurrences after conventional surgery performed without the advantage of magnification.

- Submucosal extensions of tumor are more likely to be recognized during the careful and meticulous dissection in layers around the lesion. Tumor extensions are often encountered during dissection under maximal magnification of the operating microscope. When such finger-like tumor extensions are found, this obviously necessitates a wider resection margin of another 5–10 mm.

The *safety margins* desired during laser surgery are, in principle, the same as those required for conventional surgery (e.g., partial laryngopharyngectomy). Based on our experience, we consider a safety margin of 5–10 mm on the mucosal surface adequate for resections in the hypopharynx.

A wider margin can be kept since no untoward consequences for healing and function are to be expected, even if a more liberal excision of the tumor is performed in the hypopharynx. A few millimeters more or less are of no importance, except for the area around the arytenoid cartilage.

After the incision through mucosa and submucosa has reached a depth of a few millimeters, the edge of the mucosa can be held with a small grasping forceps and pulled medially or laterally with the left hand.

In general, a certain tension should be kept on the tissue during lasering. The cut will be more precise and more effective and less tissue will be sacrificed in the process.

The example of an operation on an ulcerating tumor of the medial, anterior, and lateral wall of the pyriform sinus (Fig. 3.**43b**) will now be discussed in more detail. The procedure starts on the lateral wall of the pyriform fossa, a distance of 5–10 mm is kept from the tumor.

Submucosal tangential dissection toward the tumor must be avoided. There is a real danger that a margin which was sufficiently wide on the mucosal surface is no longer adequate in the deeper parts of the wound (Fig. 3.**3**).

If an adequate safety margin is kept, initially no tumor can be seen during the dissection. Only once the tumor is incised can the deep extension of the tumor be seen by identifying normal tissue below it. Now the resection can proceed basally into a layer of healthy tissue and an adequate margin of 5–10 mm can be maintained. The resection continues with similar incisions on the anterior and the medial wall.

If the tumor (Fig. 3.**43c**) extends further into the depth of the pyriform sinus, the initial procedure is as described. Horizontal cuts are made through the tumor in order to remove the superior parts of the lesion. The distending laryngopharyngoscope is then advanced for the further resection. The steps of the operation are repeated until the tumor is completely resected from the apex of the pyriform sinus.

If the entire pyriform sinus is filled with tumor, it is advisable to debulk the exophytic tumor in some areas to gain a better view (Fig. 3.**5**). Furthermore, the tissue can only be grasped and retracted into the lumen if there is enough space. This debulking is only necessary in cases of obstructive tumors with exophytic growth and definite deep extension (Fig. 3.**4c**) . It makes the dissection easier, clearer, and safer.

This technique of cutting through tumor during the resection and removing the tumor blockwise has a distinct advantage. It allows the surgeon to inspect the sections through the tissues, which is usually only seen by the pathologist during sectioning of the specimen (Fig. 3.**16**). With this technique the depth of infiltration of the tumor can be judged intraoperatively under the microscope and a safe margin chosen at an adequate distance from the visible edge of the tumor. If the dissection gets too close to the tumor, the margin can immediately be made wider; if there are still doubts regarding the adequacy of the resection, an additional specimen can be resected and sent for a frozen section. It is important that the pathologist should be given representative specimens for frozen section.

The surgeon must keep record in the form of a drawing of every resected tissue piece sent to the pathologist. Only then is a postoperative topographical correlation possible of clinical and histological findings. The pathologist can determine the depth of infiltration and the distance from the resection margin on every individual specimen. As usual the grade of differentiation is assessed. It is not always possible to comment on the lateral margins. If the surgeon has doubts about the lateral margin, a further specimen should be resected for either frozen-section or definitive histological examination. As one gains experience with the microsurgical technique, the necessity for these additional resections diminishes. However, it is up to the individual surgeon to obtain proof by taking representative specimens from all lateral margins and submitting them for histological examination.

As mentioned above, when using newer-generation CO_2 lasers, the degree of carbonization is determined by the tissue being cut; normal tissue showing little or none of this effect. The appearance is due to the *tissue density* and is also seen in scar tissue, severely inflamed vascular, and glandular tissue. However, these tissues are not carbonized as markedly and characteristically as tumor tissue.

These changes are particularly prominent in the hypopharynx. The cut edges of healthy tissue retract notably and the laser beam quickly reaches deeper layers. When tumor is incised, a certain "resistance" against the laser cutting is encountered in addition to carbonization.

In summary, it can be said that tumor and normal tissue can be particularly well differentiated in the hypopharynx. A relatively wide resection margin can be kept in this area without major functional consequences resulting from the additional loss of tissue. This translates into better safety for tumor resection.

General Surgical Principles

The Tumor is followed according to its superficial and deep extension and is resected with an adequate safety margin. Difficulties or limitations of this surgical technique can be met with in certain areas, such as the pyriform sinus (Table 3.**3**)

Problem Area of Lateral Wall of the Pyriform Sinus

Larger vessels can be entered into during the dissection of deeply infiltrating tumors in the lateral wall of the pyriform sinus.

Such infiltration of the soft tissues of the neck can usually be recognized preoperatively on the CT or MRI. The surgeon must take appropriate care during surgery with these cases or alternatively open the neck prophylactically to ligate the external carotid artery in order to prevent a major life-threatening hemorrhage. This is recommended by Kim Davis (Salt Lake City) for hypopharyngeal lesions. In our practice we are guided by the preoperative and intraoperative findings. In only a few cases has an intraoperative severe hemorrhage necessitated the packing of the lateral wall of oropharynx or hypopharynx and subsequent opening of the neck to ligate a vessel. This has occurred more frequently in patients with previous irradiation.

The following factors can be hazardous:

– Failure to appreciate the lateral extent of one's resection with danger of bleeding from large vessels.
– Failure to appreciate the lateral extension of the tumor into the neck due to the medial retraction during laser dissection.

Problem Area of Medial Wall of the Pyriform Sinus (Area of Arytenoid and Cricoid Cartilage)

Superficial Tumor (with or without Spread to Anterior Wall)

If the tumor does not infiltrate deeply toward the larynx (area of arytenoid and cricoid cartilage), it is dissected off the medial laryngeal wall in a cranio-caudal direction. Laryngeal structures such as false cord, arytenoid cartilage, and cricoid cartilage and as much as possible of the medial wall of the larynx are thereby preserved. This usually implies that the function of the arytenoid cartilage can be spared. The same procedure is used for carcinomas of the aryepiglottic fold (Fig. 3.**44**).

Unless the aryepiglottic fold is invaded by tumor, it need not be resected, as the extent of the resection is determined by the extension of the tumor and does not follow rigid anatomical lines. The resection in these cases is basically an extended mucosectomy of the medial wall of the pyriform sinus (Fig. 3.**43a**). The swallowing function is not impaired if the arytenoid cartilage and large parts of the supraglottic soft tissues can be spared, since the sphincter function of the larynx will be unchanged in these cases.

This is the only region of the hypopharynx where a relatively narrow margin may be kept. This is often necessitated by the careful peeling of mucosa from the lateral aspect of the arytenoid cartilage in order to preserve its function. The histological verification of the completeness of the resection is, however, still possible in this delicate area especially for superficial excisions.

The cricoarytenoid joint is a critical area. It is important to make certain that the joint has not already been invaded by tumor. This possibility must be suspected when decreased mobility of the arytenoid cartilage has been noted preoperatively. The tumor can, however, infiltrate into the joint, without evidence of reduced cord mobility.

The dissection should be performed under highest magnification of the operating microscope and low laser power. In general safe tumor resection has priority over preservation of function.

Unilateral arytenoidectomy usually only leads to temporary aspiration problems.

Infiltrating Tumor

Pointers:

– Preoperative suspicion based on decreased mobility or fixation of the arytenoid cartilage.
– Suspicion raised by radiological findings on CT and MRI.
– Intraoperatively recognizable submucosal tumor extension.

If there is a suspicion of deeply infiltrating growth of a tumor of the medial wall of the pyriform sinus, the surgical procedure is slightly modified. An initial exploratory incision is made transversely in front of the arytenoid cartilage in order to identify the depth of infiltration of the tumor (Fig. 3.**43d**).

Steps for cases of little infiltration:

– The dissection is continued along the arytenoid cartilage posteriorly and inferiorly.
– The tumor can be completely resected even with narrow margins and the arytenoid cartilage spared.

Steps for massive infiltration:

– The arytenoid cartilage is removed and the cricoid cartilage exposed.
– If the cricoid cartilage is not invaded by tumor, the dissection continues along the cartilage until the tumor has been completely resected.
– If infiltration of the cricoid can be clearly seen intraoperatively (either superficial, showing early erosion, or deep, with more extensive destruction), a partial resection of the cartilage is attempted and the resection continued until complete tumor clearance has been achieved.

In rare situations of extensive tumor spread or if the exposure is difficult, an external approach through the neck combined with an endolaryngeal approach is performed.

Unilateral infiltration of the cricoid cartilage is not necessarily a reason for total laryngectomy.

Table 3.3   Problem areas for resection in the pyriform sinus

Lateral	Soft tissues of the neck (vascular bundle–hemorrhages)
Medial	Area of cricoid and arytenoid cartilages (postoperative aspiration due to impaired function of laryngeal sphincter)
Inferior	Esophagus (stenosis with resulting dysphagia) Mediastinum (Risk of perforation with resulting descending infection and mediastinitis)

Problems with the Caudal Region of the Pyriform Sinus

Tumor can grow close to or even into the esophageal inlet. There are two different ways of spread:
– Only on the mucosal surface,
– Submucosal spread (paraesophageal).

If the extent of the tumor requires deep resection in an inferior direction, there is an ever-increasing risk of entering the mediastinum.

In this rare situation descending infection may ensue and finally result in mediastinitis. Fortunately, we have never experienced such a complication in our department.

Good exposure of the postcricoid area and the esophageal inlet with a distending laryngopharyngoscope is of paramount importance. This provides better topographical orientation, especially with regard to the actual inferior extent of the resection.

In order to avoid this complication, dissection in the caudal area of the pyriform sinus, where further inferior tumor spread is suspected, should be avoided. In this area it is also not possible to resect the specimens with a safe margin allowing for the histological confirmation of complete tumor removal.

In these situations we vaporize the tumor until tumor-free tissue becomes visible under the microscope at highest magnification. We subsequently vaporize another few millimeters of tissue to be on the safe side.

Excision around the lesion as in all the other areas of the pyriform sinus is thus not possible in this region. A resection with a very narrow margin can become necessary in this area, although this is undesirable. If the *esophageal inlet is invaded*, a few centimeters of the superior esophagus may be included in the resection if this is necessary. However, if more than half of the circumference has to be resected, there is a high risk of secondary stenosis from scarring, which might have functional implications. If even more of the esophageal mucosa needs to be resected, a large bore gastric tube (or two) should be left in as a stent for 3–4 weeks.

The feeding tube should be inserted under direct control by the surgeon through the distending laryngopharyngoscope at the end of the operation. Forced advancement of the tube without visual control carries the risk of a perforation into the mediastinum.

It must be noted that from an oncological viewpoint a slight stenosis of the esophageal inlet with preservation of the larynx is acceptable in these patients, who have a generally poor overall prognosis. This is especially so in view of the two treatment alternatives, namely radiochemotherapy for residual tumor or laryngopharyngectomy with resection of cranial esophagus and reconstruction with a jejunum interposition.

Special Situation: Invasion of the Thyroid Cartilage

It is usually quite easy to distinguish intraoperatively between the following situations:
a. Tumor reaches onto the perichondrium
b. Tumor infiltrates the perichondrium
c. Tumor infiltrates the thyroid cartilage
d. Destruction of cartilage with break-through of tumor

Surgical Steps for a and b

The dissection follows along the thyroid cartilage, which is "sterilized" on the surface with the laser beam as the operation proceeds. The advantage is improved healing and more oncological safety. In our clinical experience, there have been no recurrences within the cartilage and complications such as perichondritis or cartilage necrosis have been very rare.

The dissection along the thyroid cartilage can be performed in the conventional way with micro-instruments or with the tip of the suction. The perichondrium can usually be peeled off easily. This may be necessary where optimal histological documentation is required for the complete, however close, resection with clear margins. The resection with the laser has also been shown to allow a reliable assessment of the margins, provided there is a distance of at least 0.5–1 mm between tumor and resection line.

Surgical Steps for c and d

The *cartilage is included in the resection* and the extralaryngopharyngeal tumor extensions are resected as far as necessary and possible. Covering of the defect and reconstruction is generally not necessary. A higher power of the CO_2 laser is chosen for the transection of cartilage. If the resected cartilage (with tumor) needs to be examined histologically, the dissection should preferably be performed with laser and conventional instruments. After cutting with the laser around the lesion, cartilage pieces can be "broken out" with a large grasping forceps. Due to the tangential laser beam at microlaryngoscopy, the cartilage must be manipulated with instruments, for example, sucker or grasping forceps in order to expose or sublux it for an adequate resection.

There are some disadvantages of only using the laser for the resection of cartilage or bone with high power:
– Small flashes occur in the area of the cartilage.
– Less tissue is available for histological examination. The width of the cut and the thermal damage to the surrounding tissue is significantly greater than for laser cuts through soft tissue.
– The laser beam can hit extralaryngeal vessels through bone trabeculae. The resulting deep hemorrhage may be difficult to control.

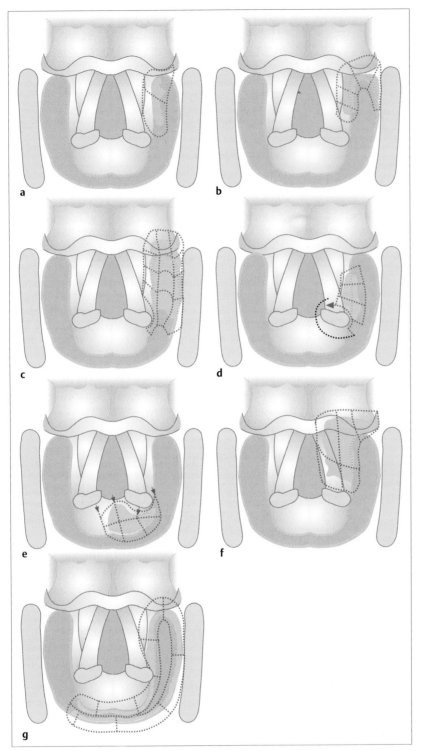

Fig. 3.43 The resection lines for hypopharyngeal carcinomas of different sites and extents are shown. **a** Carcinoma of the medial wall of the pyriform sinus. **b** Infiltration of the superior aspect of medial, anterior, and lateral wall of the pyriform sinus. **c** The right pyriform sinus is almost completely filled with a carcinoma that has grown circumferentially. **d** Carcinoma of the medial wall of the pyriform sinus with suspicion of infiltration into the larynx in the area of the arytenoid cartilage. Before the entire arytenoid cartilage is excised along its base on the cricoid cartilage, an exploratory incision is made in order to assess the depth of infiltration in the region of the arytenoid (curved arrow).**e** Carcinoma of the postcricoid. **f** Carcinoma of the right pyriform sinus with invasion of larynx and oropharynx. **g** Extensive hypopharyngeal carcinoma with progression from the right pyriform sinus toward the postcricoid and the posterior wall of the hypopharynx.

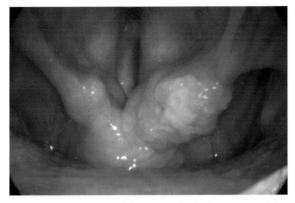
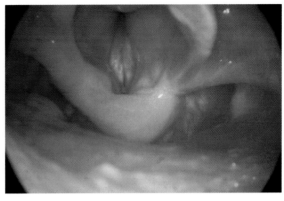

Fig. 3.**44** Carcinoma of the aryepiglottic fold on the right. The arytenoid cartilage is involved. **a** Preoperative findings. (endoscopic view, 90° telescope) **b** After transoral laser resection and adjuvant radiotherapy (1979) (N0 neck). A complete closure of the glottis is possible.

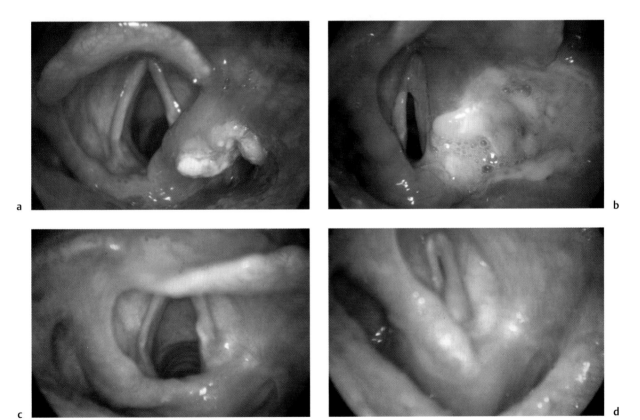

Fig. 3.**45** Pretherapeutic and posttherapeutic documentation in a carcinoma of the pyriform sinus. **a** Preoperative finding of tumor invasion into the medial and anterior wall of the pyriform sinus and to a lesser extent into the lateral wall. **b** One week after laser resection the fibrinous cover of the wound in pyriform sinus and larynx can be seen. **c** and **d** The postoperative endoscopic findings (90° telescope) during inspiration and phonation. The ipsilateral selective neck dissection showed a disease-free neck (pN0). The patient has been symptomless and tumor-free for 14 years.

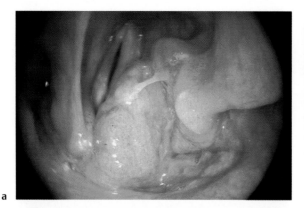

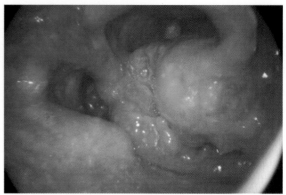

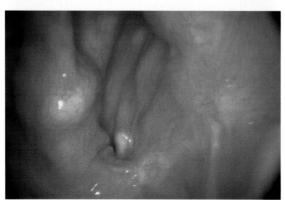

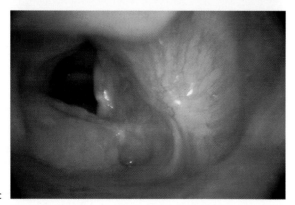

Fig. 3.**47**   Carcinoma of the postcricoid with infiltration of the interarytenoid region and both arytenoid cartilages (endoscopic view, 90° telescope). The right arytenoid is fixed, the one on the left has reduced mobility. This is a contraindication for transoral microsurgery with the laser, although it is technically quite possible. It would result in such severe aspiration that a partial laser resection would have no functional advantage.

> If deep infiltration of a tumor of the posterior wall is suspected preoperatively, a lateral radiograph of the cervical spine should be obtained, or preferably a CT scan. Invasion into the vertebral bodies can thus be excluded.

Infiltration of the prevertebral musculature and the anterior longitudinal ligament is not a technical contraindication for a transoral laser resection. Although unusual, a severe complication can, however, arise from this in the form of an abscess of the vertebral bodies and the epidural space. We have encountered one such case.

In all hypopharyngeal tumors *spontaneous healing* with complete epithelization of the wound occurs after their resection. Healing is usually complete by 4–6 weeks with very good functional results (Fig. 3.**45**).

Fig. 3.**46**   Hypopharyngeal carcinoma with infiltration of the right larynx **a** before, **b** after transoral laser microsurgical partial resection of the larynx and hypopharynx without tracheotomy. No persisting aspiration even if the arytenoid cartilage was removed (endoscopic view, 90° telescope)

Carcinomas of the Postcricoid and the Posterior Wall of the Hypopharynx

Lesions limited to the postcricoid and the posterior hypopharyngeal wall are relatively rare in Germany compared with carcinomas localized in the pyriform sinus. The microsurgical removal of tumors in both these areas is usually not a problem, provided a good exposure is obtained through the distending laryngopharyngoscope for a safe resection (Fig. 3.**43e**).

Involvement of Several Subsites (Pyriform Sinus, Postcricoid, Posterior Wall) and/or Neighboring Sites (Oropharynx, Larynx, Esophagus) (Fig. 3.43f and g)

Concomitant involvement of neighboring structures, regardless of whether it is soft tissues or cartilage, does not preclude a laser resection if no severe postoperative aspiration is to be expected. As previously mentioned, the limits of the transoral approach are reached from a technical point as soon as massive tumor infiltration into the soft tissues of the neck is present.

Postoperative Complications

There are two problems that have to be considered after the resection of very extensive tumors: Stenosis and aspiration.

A *stenosis* has to be expected if no or only very little mucosa could be preserved during the surgery for a circumferential tumor of the hypopharynx. The special problems arising from tumor involvement of the esophageal inlet have already been discussed. From a technical point of view the entire hypopharynx can be excised in its circumference. In some of our patients with very extensive circumferential tumors or recurrences after irradiation, a satisfactory result could still be achieved after such a resection. This was in spite of a stenosis in the lower hypopharynx or esophageal inlet that had formed after almost complete circumferential resection of mucosa and soft tissues in the hypopharynx with preservation of only approximately 1 cm of mucosa in one pyriform sinus. These patients were able to take a soft diet without aspiration and their laryngeal function was spared. In one patient who had suffered a circumferential recurrence after radiotherapy, regular dilatations under topical anesthesia in 2–3-monthly intervals were required. Usually, patients who are aware of the surgical alternatives will easily tolerate a slight to moderate impairment of their swallowing function and even comply with intermittent dilatations. By sparing their laryngeal function and avoiding a tracheotomy, these patients, who have a very unfavorable prognosis, can at least be provided with an improved quality of life.

Severe swallowing problems and especially *aspiration* can occur if extensive invasion of the larynx necessitates the resection of functionally important laryngeal structures. If the aryepiglottic fold and the arytenoid cartilage have to be removed along with a complete resection of the pyriform sinus, only a temporary swallowing problem is to be expected. However, if the entire pyriform sinus together with three-quarters of the larynx are removed, severe aspiration can be expected, especially in older patients. Such a resection includes everything above the level of the cricoid cartilage and anterior to the one arytenoid cartilage, thus comprising the entire supraglottis and half the larynx including the other arytenoid cartilage. Fortunately, such unfavorable tumor extensions are rarely encountered.

The massive infiltration of both arytenoid cartilages and the interarytenoid region is a contraindication for a curative laser resection (Fig. 3.**47**). Although the tumor can be resected completely via the transoral route, a degree of aspiration would result that is unacceptable to the patient.

Laser Microsurgery for Carcinomas of Oral Cavity and Oropharynx

With regards to the preoperative diagnostic work-up, the reader is referred to Chapter 3, p. 33ff. 84ff.

Operative Procedure

The operative steps and the histological confirmation of clear margins for early stages of cancer in this area are slightly different from those of other regions within the upper aerodigestive tract. *Small carcinomas of the tongue*, for instance, with a diameter of 5–10 mm are excised en bloc, although with a relatively wide resection margin of 5–10 mm. When the tumor is excised, care must be taken to keep an even distance from the tumor also in the deeper muscular layers. A mistake that is commonly made is the angling of the resection line toward the tumor in the deeper layers (Fig. 3.**3**).

A histologically proved clear mucosal edge is not equal to a complete resection of the tumor. The deeper layers must be included in the histological examination, since carcinomas of the tongue have the tendency for submucosal finger-like extensions into the deeper-lying tissues. Thus, in these cases a wider margin must be chosen from the beginning compared to, for example, a small glottic carcinoma, which is excised in one piece and sent to the pathologist for serial sectioning. In the case of a small tongue carcinoma, we cut slices from the laser-resected specimen under the microscope (Fig. 3.**4**). The specimen is unfolded with a forceps and representative sections are obtained from its sides, including the musculature and mucosal surfaces. These "specimens from the specimen" are marked, labeled, and their origin is meticulously recorded in graphic form. They should obviously be free of tumor. The remaining main specimen is serially sectioned by the pathologist and the depth of infiltration, tumor thickness, grade of differentiation, and basal resection margins are assessed. Tumors of more than 10 mm in diameter are processed by several sections through the tumor, depending on their size.

In the following sections a slightly different classification of the tumors of oral cavity and oropharynx is presented, which follows anatomical and tissue-specific but above all surgical-technical criteria. Initially, aspects common to all sites are discussed and subsequently the peculiarities of the individual organs are highlighted.

The following three "organ groups" are distinguished:
– Lip, floor of mouth, buccal area with retromolar trigone, palate, and posterior wall of oropharynx,
– Tonsil with lateral wall of oropharynx,
– Tongue, including base of tongue and vallecula.

Aspects Common to All Sites

In principle we select the intraoral approach, which generally provides a very good exposure of the oral cavity and the oropharynx. An exception to this might be, for example, a case of severe trismus. The patient is positioned low in a Trendelenburg position. Nasal intubation is relatively rarely required.

The areas involved by tumor are exposed with the aid of gags and tongue depressors (Fig. 1.**7**). Special instruments can be used to optimize the access to the operative site. Evacuation of the plume generated during the laser operation can be achieved by using retractors and other specialized laser instruments with integrated suction cannulas. In addition, an assistant can use a large-bore plastic sucker to keep oral cavity and pharynx smoke and plume free. As an alternative or further scavenging device, a suction catheter can be introduced transnasally into the oropharynx. The details of the operative procedure for smaller and larger tumors as well as the possibilities and limitations of the histological assessment of the completeness of the resection are discussed in Chapter 3, p. 43ff. These are independent of the histological type of the tumor (squamous cell carcinoma, verrucous carcinoma, mucoepidermoid tumor, etc.)

From a technical point of view, the laser excision of tumors of the oral cavity and the oropharynx is unproblematic. In cases of marked trismus, the opening of the mouth could be enlarged surgically by a maxillofacial surgeon. This is, however, rarely necessary.

Tumors with a maximum diameter of 10 mm and without evidence of deep infiltration are generally excised with a margin of approximately 5 mm. Exceptions to this are carcinomas of the tongue and tonsil. If the surface extension of the tumor is more than 10 mm or if there are indications of deep infiltration, one or more cuts are made through the tumor, depending on its localization and extent. The reliability of the assessment of the basal resection margin is thereby the decisive factor. If there are any doubts about the margins, we liberally take additional specimens from the margins in order to obtain representative tissue. We do not use punch biopsies, as these are only random samples and harbor a substantial risk for false negative results.

The surgical management of *hemorrhages* in oral cavity and oropharynx differs slightly from that in, for example, the larynx. Small bleeding points can be controlled intraoperatively and postoperatively with the bipolar electrocautery, if necessary under local anesthesia. Larger venous or arterial hemorrhages can be managed by ligation during the operation and even in the postoperative phase. Vascular clips are used less frequently in this area compared to their more frequent use through the laryngoscope in larynx and hypopharynx. The wound area where the vessel has been ligated is covered with collagen mesh and fibrin glue. Antibiotics are administered and nasogastric tube feeds are given for a few days. A transcervical approach to ligate larger vessels such as the external carotid artery is only very rarely necessary.

☞ There are some aspects of carcinogenesis and behavior of cancers that are common to oral cavity and oropharynx. Obviously the most important factors are the use of tobacco and excessive alcohol consumption, leading to the effect of field cancerization. Synchronous and metachronous second primary tumors are thus particularly common on this diffusely predamaged mucosa. There is also a relatively high rate of recurrences.

We differentiate between recurrence from the depth (e.g., submucosal extensions of a tongue carcinoma), which is caused by residual tumor or tumor cell nests, and superficial recurrence. The latter is likely due to carcinomatous changes which are difficult or impossible to identify in the mucosa next to the resection line despite the use of the

microscope. Considering the pathogenesis of squamous cell carcinoma, *field cancerization of the mucosa* must be expected particularly in patients with ethanol abuse. Severe dysplasia and carcinoma in situ occur quite frequently and are usually not recognized clinically. This not only applies to the oral cavity, but particularly also to the other areas that commonly harbor a second primary tumor, such as hypopharynx, esophagus, and bronchi. There is a strong tendency for a synchronous or metachronous second primary lesion within the upper aerodigestive tract in patients with carcinomas of the oral cavity or the oropharynx.

Another characteristic of carcinomas of the oral cavity and oropharynx is the *higher rate of local and distant metastases*. Tumors that infiltrate to a depth of only a few millimeters and that might therefore still be classified as early carcinomas can be the origin of clinically occult, clinically evident, or even advanced cervical metastases at a very early stage.

In the following sections the particularities of the different regions lip, floor of mouth, cheek, palate, and posterior wall of oropharynx are detailed with regards to oncology, operative risks, healing, function, and postoperative feeding. Borderline situations, their recognition, avoidance, and management are also discussed.

Carcinomas of the Lip

Any tumor in the region of the lip can be completely resected with the laser using the microsurgical technique and the histological processing that have already been described in detail. Limited mucosal defects need not be covered, as they usually heal spontaneously with satisfactory esthetic and functional results. Larger defects of the lips, however, unlike intraoral wounds, require reconstructive measures for esthetic reasons and even more so for functional reasons.

Carcinomas of the Floor of the Mouth

Operative Procedure

The position of the head must be adjusted several times during the operation according to the extensions of the tumor, which might extend onto the mandible or the inferior surface of the tongue. An optimal exposure can usually be achieved. From a purely technical aspect the resection of any carcinoma of the floor of the mouth is possible. The tumor is followed into the surrounding healthy tissue regardless of the direction and degree of its extension.

Two special situations deserve more detailed discussion. These are firstly the inclusion of the excretory ducts of the sublingual and submandibular glands in the resection, and secondly the modification of the procedure if involvement of the mandible is present. As previously described, the resection is performed in several pieces. This is done in order to obtain a clear view under the microscope of the border between tumor and healthy tissue in all the areas of the resection and especially in the deeper parts of the wound. If massive infiltration of the musculature of the floor of mouth is found, the resection can extend all the way into the soft tissues of the neck. The excretory ducts of the lesser salivary glands are severed or partially resected in the process. Sometimes even parts of a salivary gland are included in the resection, particularly of the sublingual gland. The large wound defects heal spontaneously by filling up with granulation tissue. Complete epithelization occurs quite rapidly (Fig. 3.**48**).

The obliteration of the excretory ducts of the smaller salivary glands can theoretically have various sequelae. It is, however, surprising how seldom we are confronted with complications such as chronic inflammation with intermittent swelling of the gland, which requires treatment and might eventually necessitate the excision of the gland. The explanation for this is firstly the fact that the excretory duct is generally preserved in cases of superficial carcinomas. On the other hand, the pressure of the saliva is usually great enough to keep the lumen patent and prevent a stenosis from forming.

Large parts of the duct system are removed during the resection of more extensive, deeply infiltrating tumors. In these cases a neck dissection is commonly performed at a later stage, during which the submandibular gland is routinely removed. If a very extensive resection has been performed, which extended deeply into the musculature of the floor of the mouth, the neck dissection is only performed after 8–10 days. This helps to avoid any through and through defect between the oral cavity and the neck wound and thus reduces the possibility of a fistula formation. So far we have had no complications in this regard within our group of patients, which is, however, rather small.

Carcinomas of the Floor of the Mouth with Extension Toward the Mandible and Invasion of the Mandible

The carcinoma can either reach onto the mandible on the mucosal surface, or involve the periosteum or already infiltrate the bone. The latter usually occurs via the empty tooth sockets. The carcinoma can even erode through the mandible. This observation has been extremely rare in our small patient population.

Operative Procedure

We excise the tumor with a safety margin of at least 5 mm. The periosteum can be dissected off with the laser or a rasp. The basal surface is marked with blue ink and is submitted for histological examination. If there is the suspicion of infiltration into the bone, the area in question is excised widely. For this purpose the laser is used in combination with conventional instruments in order to preserve as much bone tissue on the specimen as possible for the histological examination. The CO_2 laser (unlike the excimer laser) is not particularly well-suited for cutting of bone since high power is required

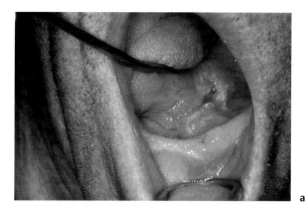

a

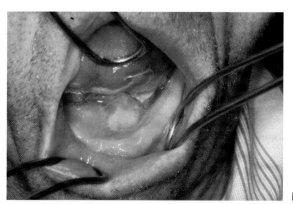

b

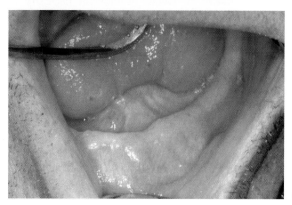

c

Fig. 3.**48**　Left-sided carcinoma of the floor of mouth with extension onto the under surface of the tongue. Preoperative and postoperative findings are documented. **a** The ulcerating tumor of the left floor of mouth stretches to the midline and extends posteriorly to involve the inferior surface of the tongue. **b** The fibrin layer and some sutures can be seen after 6 days. **c** Completely healed scar in the left floor of mouth without any signs of recurrence.

for this purpose, resulting in small sparks and flames, which are irritating and distracting for the surgeon. If a lower power setting is chosen, the operation takes significantly longer. A further aspect is the heat developing in the surrounding tissue, which is much greater than for the transection of mucosa. Although this heat may kill tumor cells, its effects lead to an impairment of the histological examination. For this reason we complete the partial resection of the mandible with an osteotome or the oscillating saw after initial laser dissection of the soft tissues. Subsequent to the resection of the bone segment, the entire area of exposed bone is treated superficially with the laser.

☞ In our opinion it is not the cutting instrument that is important but the oncological concept of the procedure. We always attempt to primarily perform marginal resections of the mandible and thus preserve the continuity of the bone (Fig. 3.**49**).

In our small group of patients we have managed to achieve very good long-term results, both oncological and functional, after marginal resection of the mandible. We leave the bone to heal spontaneously regardless of whether it is covered by periosteum, cancellous bone has been resected, or the marrow spaces have been entered into. During the operation, the bone is not covered by mucosa, tongue or skin flaps, or any other soft tissue. Patients are treated with antibiotics for 8–10 days and are encouraged to rinse their mouth with an antiseptic solution several times per day.

Wound healing of the soft tissue in the floor of mouth is complete after 3–4 weeks, depending on the size of the defect. The healing of the bone can take several months and is especially delayed by preoperative or postoperative irradiation to the area. Occasionally, small bony sequestra are expelled from the wound in the course of the wound healing. The necessity for additional laser treatment to the wound arises only on rare occasions. It could be shown that the CO_2 laser has a *sterilizing effect* also on osseous structures. The final results are very satisfactory with regard to wound healing, although this might be delayed slightly (Fig. 3.**49**).

A decisive factor for the final result is always the *compliance of the patient*. In patients who continue to smoke, drink large quantities of alcohol, and neglect their oral hygiene, poor and protracted wound healing can become a problem. Patients with extensive wound surfaces in the floor of the mouth and the under surface of the tongue are encouraged to perform regular and frequent *exercises with the tongue*. Lifting of the tongue and regular movement help prevent adhesions between the floor of mouth and the tongue. This is what we have experienced during the follow-up of patients who underwent a secondary operation to mobilize the tongue with the CO_2 laser after initial conventional surgery. In these patients the tongue is sutured into the defect in the floor of mouth and later loosened again. We have used the laser for this secondary dissection and discovered that active tongue movements helped to prevent the formation of further adhesions.

Another important factor is *nutrition in the postoperative period*. The size of the wound defect is also of importance. In cases of small wounds, the patient can be started on an oral diet, especially fluids, as early as day 1–2 after the surgery. An enteral feeding tube is not required. From day 3 a soft diet can be fed to patients, who must obviously rinse their mouth regularly after meals. If there are larger defects in the area of floor of mouth and tongue area, a nasogastric feeding tube is recommended for a few days. These patients can start on a liquid diet on day 4–5 and after 8 days a soft diet can be introduced. The prerequisite for the feeding of these patients is the formation of a thin layer of granulation tissue. This will prevent food particles from collecting in the wound, causing a subsequent infection. Early feeding can even provide an additional stimulus for the formation of granulation tissue. In any case and despite open wounds, the patients can begin to drink clear fluids at a very early stage.

Carcinomas of Buccal Mucosa, Oral Surface of Soft and Hard Palate and Uvula

Superficial and exophytic *carcinomas of the buccal mucosa* which do not break through the skin of the cheek or infiltrate the parotid gland can be completely resected with the laser and a microsurgical technique. Reconstruction of the defect is not necessary, as these wounds heal spontaneously and without significant functional impairment. The same that has been said about Wharton's duct in the case of the submandibular gland applies for Stenson's duct. We have so far not encountered a stenosis, although our case numbers are limited. For very extensive lesions with invasion of parotid and skin, a combined internal and external approach is advocated. In these cases it becomes necessary to repair the resulting defect with plastic-reconstructive methods.

The resection of *carcinomas of the soft palate* follows a similar pattern. The nasopharynx is protected with moist gauze swabs during this operation. So far we have not performed any reconstructions even after very extensive resections in the area of the palate. Limited defects in the bone are also not covered, as they heal spontaneously. In the case of superficially spreading carcinomas (Fig. 3.**50**), it is usually possible to preserve a muscle layer with the posterior mucosa, thus preventing a through and through defect. Massive infiltration of the hard palate has been an extremely rare finding in our patient population. However, it can happen that a large portion of the soft palate has to be resected. In such a case an initial velopalatal incompetence can be observed. Fluids and food may escape from the nose during swallowing and the patient tends to speak through his nose. In the course of the wound healing, however, a more or less marked scar formation results in some form of stenosis in the area of the oropharynx (Fig. 3.**51** and 3.**52**). This velopalatal incompetence during swallowing has not therefore persisted in any of our patients. It was never necessary to reconstruct the palate with a flap. A resection of the entire soft palate and large parts of the hard palate is an exception at least in our patient population. In the exceptional case where functional problems, including nasal speech, persist, the patient can either be managed with a dental prosthesis of extra length or the closure of the defect with a flap might be considered. The reconstruction in

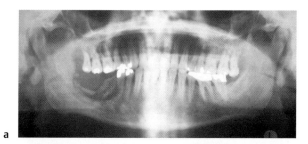

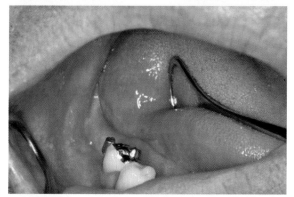

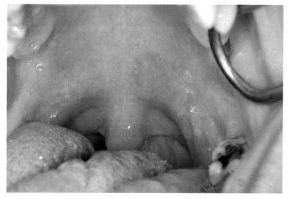

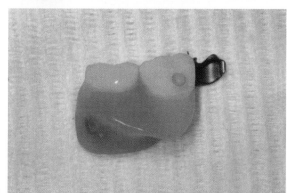

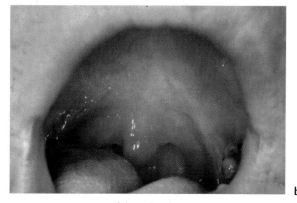

Fig. 3.**50** Carcinoma of the soft palate on the left side before and after laser resection. a Preoperative finding. The tumor reaches the midline and spreads in the area of the ipsilateral tonsil. It is a superficial lesion with areas of erythroplakia and ulceration. b The findings after laser excision show a discrete, fine line of whitish scar tissue.

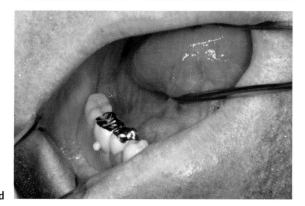

Fig. 3.**49** Findings after resection of a carcinoma of the retromolar trigone with invasion of the floor of mouth and infiltration of the mandible posteriorly. **a** The orthopantomogram shows the bony defect in the mandible. **b** The scar after full healing has taken place. The wound was left to heal spontaneously and was not covered. **c** Dental prosthesis. **d** Prosthesis in place.

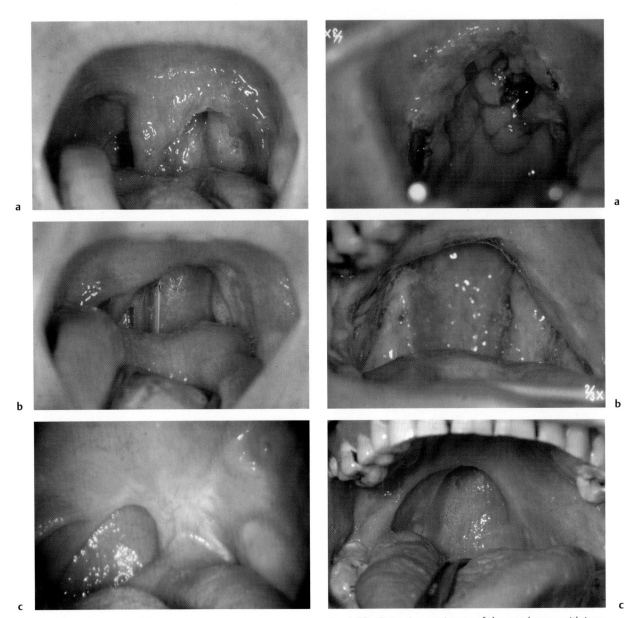

Fig. 3.**51** Carcinoma of the oropharynx.
a The preoperative findings were that of involvement of uvula, soft palate, and the entire tonsillar region on the left with extension onto the posterior wall of the oropharynx.
b A fibrinous exudate can be seen in the wound area 1 week after laser resection.
c Five months after the operation with the laser surprisingly marked scar formation has taken place stretching up to the nasopharynx. A relatively small opening is left, however, without functional effects for the patient. We did not pursue any reconstruction or fitting of a prosthesis postoperatively because of the satisfactory functional result.

Fig. 3.**52** Extensive carcinoma of the oropharynx with invasion of soft palate, uvula, both tonsils, and the posterior wall of the oropharynx bilaterally.
a Preoperative findings.
b A few weeks after laser resection, there is a fibrinous membrane on both sides in the area of the resection.
c Findings at 10 months after laser operation and adjuvant radiotherapy. The patient had no clinically detectable cervical metastases and no neck dissection was performed, since postoperative irradiation had been planned. The patient has now been free of tumor for 12 years and is highly satisfied with the functional result.

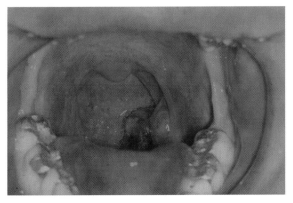

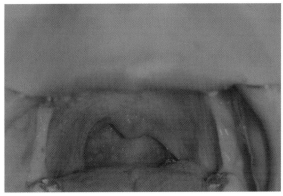

a

b

Fig. 3.**53** Tonsillar carcinoma on the left side in a young woman. **a** The exophytic tumor can be seen before the laser resection. Several metastases were found in the specimen from the ipsilateral selective neck dissection. **b** Findings after intraoral laser resection. The patient did not have postoperative radiotherapy and has been disease-free for more than 18 years.

these cases is best performed with the help of a free radial forearm flap.

In carcinomas of the palate as well as tonsillar carcinomas, the possibility of an extension into the nasopharynx must be considered. The tumor can spread superficially onto the posterior aspect of the soft palate or there might even be a second primary in this region. From this arises the necessity for preoperative and intraoperative endoscopic assessment of the entire region.

Carcinomas of the Posterior Wall of the Oropharynx

Technically the tumors of the posterior wall can be completely resected without any difficulties. If there is tumor extension toward the hypopharynx or nasopharynx, the resection is extended accordingly.

The superior extent can usually be adequately exposed with the help of palatal retractors. Transpalatal approach with temporary splitting of the soft palate is only rarely required to improve the exposure. The distending laryngopharyngoscope is used for cases with significant inferior extent.

Cases of deeply infiltrating tumors of the posterior wall of the oropharynx are managed similar to those of the hypopharynx. The latter have been discussed in Chapter 3, p. 90ff.

Wounds in this area *heal* very well and again without the need to cover the defect. As a matter of fact, limited defects heal so well that one has difficulties in finding the operated site during postoperative endoscopic examinations. In some of our patients very extensive resections were necessary from the nasopharynx to the esophageal inlet. These large wound surfaces with a significant depth also healed spontaneously.

A certain stiffness of the posterior pharyngeal wall does, however, result and is caused by scar formation. The passage of food during swallowing is also at least temporarily affected. Due to the loss of sensation of the mucosa of the posterior wall, these patients experience some difficulties with swallowing of food. Nevertheless, in general there are no persisting problems of great significance.

Carcinomas of the Lateral Wall of the Oropharynx: Tonsil, Glossotonsillar Groove, Palatal Arches

The surgical and histological procedures for carcinomas of the tonsil differ from those for other regions. The different tissue structure and growth characteristics of the tumors in this area necessitate a modification of the surgical approach and the histological confirmation of a complete resection.

Well-circumscribed lesions with a more superficial growth pattern and a size of 5–10 mm would be excised en bloc if they occurred in any of the regions that have so far been discussed. They would then be serially sectioned and completely analyzed histologically similar to a carcinoma of the vocal cord. However, for the early stage of a tonsillar carcinoma the minimum excision is *at least a tonsillectomy* (Fig. 3.**53**). The true early stages of tonsil carcinomas are found at tonsillectomy, which is performed as part of the search for an unknown primary tumor in patients presenting with a cervical metastasis. These tumors grow submucosally and are commonly microcarcinomas. Clinically the tonsils do not give rise to any suspicion and the microcarcinoma within the tonsil is only discovered at histological examination by serial sectioning.

Larger tumors in the area of the tonsil are resected in several pieces as previously described. We perform at least three horizontal incisions: one superiorly, one

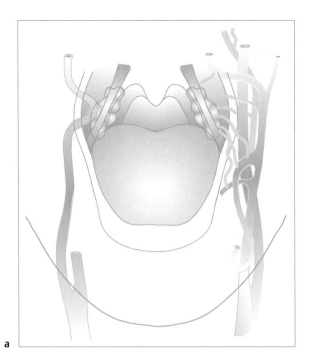

a

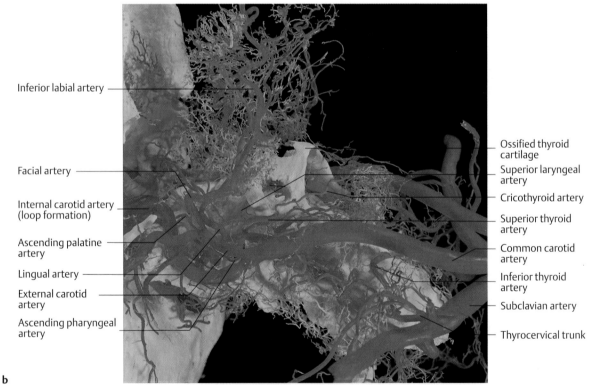

Inferior labial artery

Facial artery

Internal carotid artery
(loop formation)

Ascending palatine
artery

Lingual artery

External carotid
artery

Ascending pharyngeal
artery

Ossified thyroid
cartilage

Superior laryngeal
artery

Cricothyroid artery

Superior thyroid
artery

Common carotid
artery

Inferior thyroid
artery

Subclavian artery

Thyrocervical trunk

b

Fig. 3.**54**   Limitations and risks of intraoral resections of oropharyngeal and especially tonsillar carcinomas. Knowledge of
the anatomy of the large vessels and their relation to the
affected and operated region is one of the most important
prerequisites to avoid severe intraoperative and postoperative
complications. We are currently working on an illustration of
these anatomical relations from a transendoscopic aspect
which is more practical and useful for the surgeon. **a** The drawing demonstrates the close proximity of the great vessels and
illustrates the limits of the intraoral operation. An abnormal
course of the internal carotid artery is shown on the left side of
the picture. In rare instances the vessel can reach to within a
few millimeters of the tonsillar capsule. **b** Corrosion specimen
of the arteries of the head and neck with intact skeletal
structures of a 79-year-old male. This specimen is part of the
collection of the Institute of Anatomy at the Christian
Albrechts University in Kiel, Germany (Director: Professor
B. Tillmann, specimen by G.-R. Klaws, photo by B. Tillmann).

through the middle, and one inferiorly. It is of particular importance in the tonsillar area to recognize the deep extension of the tumor during the operation. Since the close proximity of the great vessels sets a limit for the lateral extent of the resection, extensive carcinomas of the tonsil (Fig. 3.**54**) should be investigated preoperatively with CT or MRI.

If there is superficial spread of the tumor into floor of mouth and tongue or vallecula and hypopharynx, the resection must be extended accordingly. A critical situation arises if the tumor spreads to involve the area around the eustachian tube orifice. This is, however, a rather rare occurrence. In this area the soft tissues can also be resected with the laser under microscopic control but this is a high risk procedure, due to the proximity of the internal carotid artery. It is not possible to excise the tumor with a wide margin of healthy tissue in this region.

☞ The lymphatic tissue structure and the chronic inflammatory reaction within the tonsils make the intraoperative assessment of the tumor borders more difficult. Increased carbonization, as is characteristically observed in tumor tissue, is also caused by recent inflammation, mini-abscesses, and scars. The evaluation of the tissues during the dissection again becomes easier outside the tonsillar capsule in the pharyngeal musculature.

✄ If the dissection reaches far laterally toward the vascular bundle, greatest care must be taken in the assessment of changing tissue characteristics (connective tissue, fatty tissue, etc.) and pulsations must be looked out for.

❗ The surgeon should work under the highest magnification at very low power and proceed particularly slowly and cautiously. When the immediate proximity of the great vessels has been reached, conventional instruments, such as suction cannula and grasping forceps, should be used for the dissection and for spreading of the tissues.

If the operation is to be successfully completed from the inside, a resection onto the great vessels may become necessary. In these cases we cover the defect with collagen mesh and fibrin glue. Branches of the ascending palatine artery (from the facial artery) and of the descending palatine artery (from the maxillary artery) as well as branches of the ascending pharyngeal artery are ligated conventionally or with vascular clips.

☞ The glossotonsillar groove is also a high risk area for deeper, more extensive resections with regard to larger arterial vessels such as the lingual artery and the external carotid artery. Other important structures in the immediate proximity are the hypoglossal and glossopharyngeal nerves. Here the same safety precautions apply as do in the area lateral to the tonsil.

A special characteristic of the glossotonsillar region is the difficult exposure. Regardless of whether it is a primary tumor of the glossotonsillar groove or whether a carcinoma of the tonsil, tongue, or floor of mouth has invaded this area, good exposure remains a problem in all these cases. In order to succeed with a curative resection, a good exposure of the glossotonsillar groove can only be achieved with the aid of special self-retaining retractors, for example, otological retractors, spatulas, or the distending laryngopharyngoscope.

✄ If the tumor cannot be completely resected via the intraoral approach or if the risk for secondary hemorrhages is too great, it is recommended to open the neck and ligate the feeding vessels or even the external carotid artery in certain cases. Of course a neck dissection is performed at the same time. It is usually not necessary to cover the defect from the outside. Should this, however, become necessary, it is sufficient to swing a neck muscle into the wound area as cover.

Tongue, Base of Tongue, and Vallecula

There are a number of factors that complicate the technically simple laser resection of carcinomas of the tongue. The relatively common tumor extensions especially into the submucosal space are oncologically unfavorable characteristics of these cancers. The identification of the tumor borders is more difficult in the tongue than in the larynx. The more pronounced *char formation*, encountered during lasering of tongue tissue, is a result of the increased vascularization and of the glandular tissue present in the tongue. Already the cut through the surface of the tongue is different due to the well-vascularized tissue of high density. More carbonization than usual is encountered in this organ, making the intraoperative differentiation between tumor and normal tissue more difficult for the surgeon.

Advanced carcinomas of the tongue require the resection of more than half, in some instances even up to three quarters of the tongue. The main complication in these cases is the resulting severe functional impairment, which is fortunately of a mainly temporary nature. The following problems are encountered:

– Impaired swallowing
– Aspiration
– Unintelligible speech
– Continuous drooling.

Finally, the relatively *high rate of recurrences* must be added to this list. It is well known that even a total glossectomy with laryngectomy cannot improve the poor prognosis of advanced cancers of the tongue with cervical metastatic disease. These patients usually succumb to regional and distant metastases, second primary tumors in esophagus and bronchi, or systemic diseases caused by smoking and excessive alcohol consumption (liver cirrhosis, cardiac and lung diseases, etc.). An extensive, radical surgical procedure with reconstruction is difficult to justify ethically in these cases, especially when one considers the alternative of simultaneous radiotherapy and chemotherapy. A primary total glossectomy with the laser using a

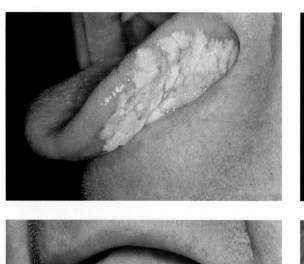

a

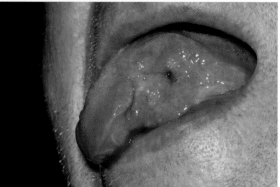

b

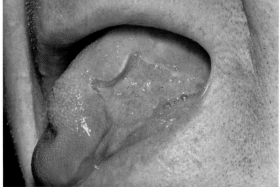

c

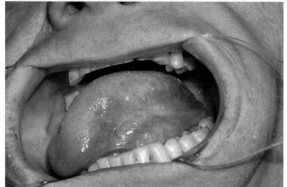

d

Fig. 3.**55** Squamous cell carcinoma of the inferior and lateral aspects of the tongue. Preoperative findings and course of treatment are shown. **a** Leukoplakia and hyperkeratosis of the left lateral edge of the tongue. **b** Postoperatively, granulation tissue has formed in the wound area. A small cauterized vessel can be seen. The wound was not closed. **c** A few weeks after the laser resection, the wound is healing. Definite granulation tissue formation can be noted. **d** Final situation after wound healing has been completed. A very satisfactory functional result was achieved in this case.

microsurgical technique does not pose great technical difficulties. However, in view of the unfavorable overall prognosis of these cases, I have so far not been able to recommend this to any patient.

In the past we have encountered patients who explicitly requested several operations for local recurrences and who ended up with an almost complete resection of tongue and floor-of-mouth musculature. These patients managed to adjust their swallowing technique surprisingly well and could thus be spared a laryngectomy. This has, however, been observed in only few, mainly young patients, who explicitly preferred to undergo further surgery rather than receive any other form of palliative treatment. These patients finally died of tumor cachexia from an uncontrolled primary tumor and after nearly total removal of tongue and floor of mouth, although there was no evidence of regional recurrence, distant metastases, or a second primary tumor.

Hemostasis is achieved as usual in the oral cavity, if necessary with the bipolar electrocautery or a suction diathermy. Larger vessels can be ligated. The wound edges are approximated with sutures for a few days to prevent secondary bleeding and infections and in order to make oral feeding possible at a very early stage (first postoperative day). The sutures can be removed after 5–6 days. It could be shown that wounds which granulate from within result in smaller defects and lead to a better function of the tongue (Fig. 3.**55**, 3.**56**).

Carcinomas of the Tongue Base (Fig. 3.**57**)

Operative Procedure

The surgical steps are the same as for hypopharyngeal tumors (see Chapter 3, p. 84ff.). The extremely rare tumors of small size, i.e., diameter of 5 mm are excised in one piece and can be analyzed histologically with great ease. In most cases, however, several cuts have to be made through the tumor depending on its size and localization. A minimum of two incisions that are perpendicular to each other and cross in the middle of the tumor are recommended for this.

Apart from the postcricoid region, the base of tongue is the *most unfavorable area* for endoscopic surgery, especially if the exposure through the distending laryngopharyngoscope is not optimal. Another aggravating factor is the differentiation between tumor and healthy tissue, which is particularly difficult in the area of the tongue base due to the lingual tonsil.

It can be extremely difficult to achieve adequate access to this region with sufficient exposure of all the areas that are involved by tumor. The surgeon can usually only see a certain segment and may lack any surrounding *landmarks*, such as pyriform sinus or larynx, for orientation. Throughout the operation the surgeon has continuously and exclusively the tissues of the tongue base in view, with little change in the surface structure. The only landmarks are the medial glossoepiglottic fold, the foramen caecum, and the vallecula. If the blades of the distending laryngopharyngoscope are spread too far apart, tongue tissue protrudes into the lumen from the side and can lead to an impaired view.

| The protrusion from tissues can be prevented by the use of the distending oropharyngoscope (Fig. 1.**4**)

Practical hints:
– The intermittent assessment of the wound through the endoscope during the operation improves orientation and should always be done as a matter of routine at the end of the procedure. It is recommended to remove the oropharyngoscope for this purpose and introduce the McIntosh laryngoscope. A 30° or 70° telescope or flexible endoscope can then be inserted for inspection of the wound cavity or better orientation. ≤
– Alternatively, the tongue can be pulled out and a tongue depressor inserted, over which the telescopes are advanced toward the tongue base.
– Finally, the surgeon might want to use the gag for a tonsillectomy. This is especially useful for the exposure of the glossotonsillar groove and the area of the lateral wall of the oropharynx.
– Furthermore, digital palpation should be employed in regular intervals during the operation.
– The transoral use of ultrasound probes can be an additional aid for the identification of relatively large submucosal tumor extensions.

The operation can be difficult and demanding from a technical aspect. One common problem, for instance, is the repeated slipping of the tongue blade anteriorly toward the oral cavity during the opening of the bivalved laryngoscope.

| In these cases it can be helpful to pull the tongue anteriorly and insert the oropharyngoscope while this traction is maintained. This is particularly useful if further resections are planned in the direction of the body of the tongue. Great care must, however, be taken with this exposure and the excessive pressure must not be maintained for too long, as the teeth can be pressed into the tongue, resulting in tissue damage, postoperative pain, and functional disturbances.

Not only is the tongue base a problem area because of the difficult exposure and topographical orientation, but also due to the difficulties that are encountered in the differentiation between tumor and lingual tonsil, as has been described for tumors of the tongue. Cutting with the laser in this area can lead to increased carbo-

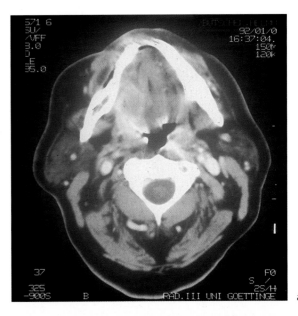

a

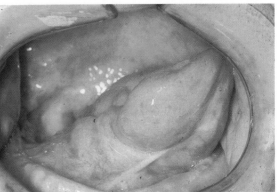

b

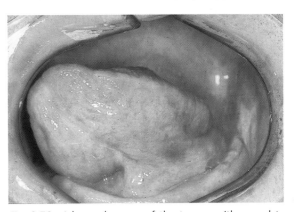

c

Fig. 3.**56** Advanced cancer of the tongue with spread to the base of the tongue and to the floor of the mouth (T3). **a** Preoperative CT scan. **b**, **c** Postoperative aspects. As the result of the spontaneous healing of the large wound without reconstructive surgery for covering the defect with flaps, the remaining tongue shows a very good functional mobility.

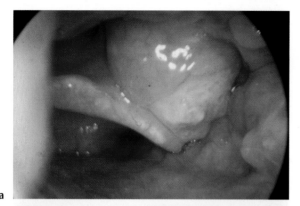

a

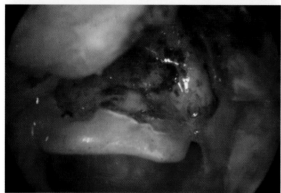

b

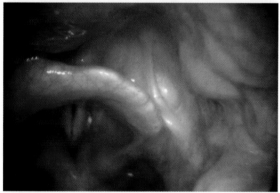

c

Fig. 3.**57**   Carcinoma of the base of tongue before and after laser resection. **a** The exophytic tumor of the left tongue base fills the vallecula and makes contact with the lingual surface of the epiglottis. **b** A few days after the laser resection a large defect is apparent in the area of the tongue base. The mucosa of the lingual surface of the epiglottis and the vallecula has been removed. **c** A few months after the operation an easily visualized defect remains in the area of the right tongue base and vallecula. No radiotherapy was given. The patient subsequently succumbed to an unrelated second malignancy in the colon.

nization caused by the higher tissue density, the increased vascularization, and the large proportion of muscle and glandular tissue. The situation is similar to that in the tonsil, which has already been discussed. Severe chronic inflammation with little necrotic cavities and abscess formations can simulate tumor tissue. Fibrosis from previous inflammatory processes in the base of tongue also leads to a different tissue reaction to the laser beam and can make the tissue assessment more difficult during lasering. If there is tumor extension anteriorly or inferiorly toward the musculature of the floor of mouth or the fat of the preepiglottic space, the resection must be extended accordingly. The operative conditions for the differentiation of tumor and healthy tissue are better in these areas than in the tongue base.

⚡ Frozen-section examinations should be employed more frequently for surgery on the tongue base.

The use of *imaging techniques* with contrast enhancement, for example MRI, can be helpful for the preoperative assessment of tumor extension and for the follow-up of the patient.

Practical hints:
– It is recommended to use low laser power of 4–6 W for the dissection through healthy tissue. The operation should proceed slowly layer by layer and avoid deep incisions at any one point resulting in "keyhole surgery."
– It is advisable rather to obtain several small specimens than to resect large blocks of tissue.
– Hemostasis must be achieved immediately and diligently as the operation proceeds.
– The cut surface should always be inspected under highest magnification of the microscope; frozen-section examination should be made use of to ensure clear surgical margins. The specimens taken must be carefully orientated and the relevant surface clearly marked. These specimens are taken in the final stages of the resection, when the major tumor bulk has been removed. This has been referred to as the "fine-tuning" of the operation.

This type of surgery is quite demanding for the surgeon. It is more time-consuming and a change of instruments is often required. The oropharyngoscope must continuously be repositioned. All this requires a lot of patience and experience on the part of the surgeon.

Finally, the *comparison of intraoperative findings with histological results* is particularly difficult as well as time-consuming but cannot and must not be dispensed with. Additional resections at a later stage can be aimed at the particular area questioned by the pathologist. The prerequisite for this is obviously an excellent and meticulous documentation of the intraoperative findings on video or alternatively with the help of a schematic drawing of the operative situation.

There is one oncologically disadvantageous quality of these cancers of the base of tongue, which they share with tumors of the tongue. This is the submucosal extension of these tumors, which can occur under a clinically perfectly intact mucosal surface. The recognition of these finger-like projections of the cancer into the surrounding tissue is of crucial importance for the correct treatment. These extensions can only be identified if representative specimens are taken from the wound cavity in all three dimensions and submitted to the pathologist for the arduous histological processing and examination.

An additional complicating factor is the possibility of *multiple foci of carcinoma*. This has already been discussed in another context. These foci can occur in the immediate vicinity of the clinically apparent tumor as carcinomatous changes in the neighboring mucosa. They might also be completely independent from the main tumor and, in the case of carcinoma in situ or microcarcinoma, may be impossible or very difficult to identify clinically. In patients who present with a cervical metastasis as main symptom (often N2a or N3) and clinically occult primary tumor, cancers are relatively often found in the tonsil or the tongue base. We were able to prove the existence of submucosal nests of tumor cells (microcarcinomas) in specimens obtained during deep and extensive laser excisions from the tongue base similar to findings in the tonsil after tonsillectomy.

These tumors were so small that they could be neither identified by clinical palpation nor by CT or MRI investigations.

Side Effects and Complications

Pain. After resections of the base of tongue, patients complain of surprisingly little pain and definitely not more pain than after a tonsillectomy. On the contrary, the pain is usually considerably less. It is thereby of no importance whether the resection has been performed for benign hyperplasia or for a carcinoma. In some patients, however, postoperative pain can occur and radiate to the ear. These neuralgia-like pains can occasionally be very severe. They might have their origin in the free-lying nerve endings after laser transection and thermal damage of, for example, fibers of the glossopharyngeal nerve.

Hemorrhages. Bleeding is more pronounced after cutting into tongue, than, for example, into the less vascularized vocal cord. More severe hemorrhages can occur when branches of the lingual artery are severed, such as the deep lingual artery, the sublingual artery, or the dorsal branches of the lingual artery. We have only rarely encountered these larger bleedings. If they occur, the vessels can be ligated or clipped. A ligation of the feeding vessels in the neck is only necessary in exceptional cases. There has been no increased tendency for secondary hemorrhages in the postoperative phase compared to tonsillectomies. No patient has succumbed to a complication.

"Increased" saliva and mucus production. This is a result of the initial impairment of the swallowing function. Patients avoid swallowing their own saliva because of pain or because of the coughing caused by the transient aspiration. This gives the impression of increased saliva production. In reality, however, it is the delay and painful impairment of the natural transport mechanism for saliva.

Functional disturbances. The bilateral transection of the hypoglossal nerves must be avoided under all circumstances during the tumor resection. A marked, although temporary, impairment of tongue mobility can occur postoperatively. Swallowing can be resumed relatively quickly if the sphincter function of the larynx (epiglottis and both arytenoid cartilages) has been preserved. Loss of sensation in the oropharyngeal mucosa after very extensive resections can be a contributory cause for swallowing problems.

Halitosis. Large wound defects in the area of the tongue base and vallecula can lead to salivary pooling and temporary retention of food. We prescribe regular mouthwashes and gargles for these patients similar to the postoperative care after a procedure in the oral cavity. Antibiotics are also administered. Prophylactic mouthwashes for the prevention of fungal infections are also an important element of the oral hygiene. Of course, the extent of the resection largely determines the above-mentioned functional disturbances and other occurring side effects. The scar formation after very extensive resections of the tongue base with parts of the floor of mouth musculature and the epiglottis can lead to the restriction of tongue protrusion from the mouth, despite retained tongue mobility.

Aftercare

Gastric feeding tube. The insertion of a PEG tube should be considered after very extensive operations which include the resection of large parts of the larynx. The insertion of a PEG tube should be made more readily if adjuvant radiotherapy and chemotherapy are planned in cases of advanced metastatic disease in the neck.

Swallowing exercises and early oral feeding. Both are stimuli for the formation of new tissue, which will fill in the wound defects in an impressive way. This rehabilitation process, which was first observed by Alonso after supraglottic laryngectomies, can also be seen after laser resections in other areas.

Follow-up

Routine follow-up comprises endoscopic assessment and regular ultrasound examination of the neck. This should be supplemented by MRI (Fig. 3.**58**) in high risk patients. In individual cases MRI can help to identify residual tumor that was left behind at operation. It is even more useful as a follow-up investigation for the detection of clinically occult submucosal recurrences and is commonly performed twice per year.

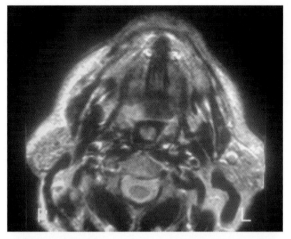

a

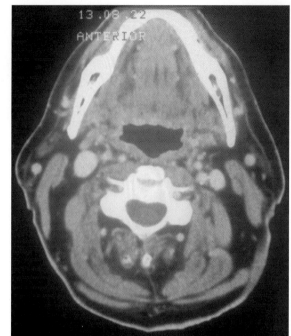

b

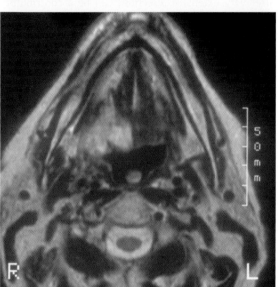

c

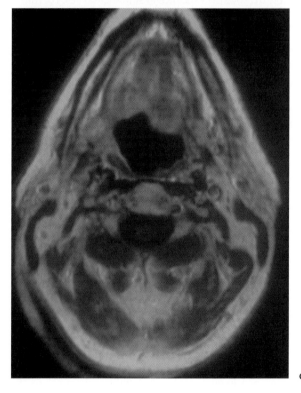

d

Fig. 3.**58**   Recurrence of a tongue base carcinoma after combined radiotherapy and chemotherapy. Imaging techniques were used to document the course of the disease. **a** Pretherapeutic finding of a relatively small carcinoma in the right tongue base (MRI image, T2 weighted). **b** A few months after combined radiotherapy and chemotherapy, no definite residual tumor can be identified in the area of the previous carcinoma in the right tongue base (contrasted CT scan). **c** Almost 2 years later an extensive tumor recurrence with small central necrosis is detected in the tongue base (intense signal on the T2 weighted MRI). **d** Two months after transoral laser resection of the recurrent cancer in the tongue base. There is a marked defect from the operation in the right tongue base. No tumor can be detected (MRI scan, T1 weighted, uncontrasted). The patient was disease-free but succumbed to a second primary tumor of the gastrointestinal tract

Palliative CO₂ Laser Surgery of Larynx, Oropharynx, and Hypopharynx

Indications: Primary tumors or recurrences leading to obstruction. The main symptom is usually respiratory distress.

Aim: To avoid a tracheotomy.

Operative procedure: Transoral debulking of the tumor with the laser using a microsurgical technique.

The palliative, symptomatic laser treatment is in general much more difficult than curative resections of laryngeal or hypopharyngeal carcinomas. Often the patients present with extensive recurrences, for example, after irradiation that have lead to breathing and swallowing problems. The difficulties encountered are usually not of a technical nature. These operations are on the contrary commonly regarded as simple and suitable to learn and practice the manual skills required for endoscopic laser surgery. What is not considered, however, is the difficulty that is encountered with this form of surgery in judging the exact extent of the resection. This again does require great experience. If too little tumor is resected, the dyspnea persists and the patient requires a tracheotomy. If too much is resected, subsequent massive aspiration can make a secondary tracheotomy necessary. In both these cases the palliative, symptomatic laser operation fails to reach its primary aim, namely an improved quality of life. The cases of two patients will be used to illustrate the surgical procedure and the resulting consequences. Both patients had a recurrence of a hypopharyngeal tumor after primary radiotherapy and suffered from breathing and swallowing difficulties.

In patient A we attempted the complete removal of the tumor. The resection included the arytenoid cartilage and extended onto the level of the cricoid cartilage. The entire pyriform sinus was removed in the process. The patient was unable to swallow postoperatively and aspirated. He required a secondary tracheotomy (Fig. 3.**59**).

In patient B tumor tissue was only removed to an extent that opened the laryngeal inlet and guaranteed a patent airway. The complete removal of the tumor was deliberately not attempted. This patient did not require a subsequent tracheotomy (Fig. 3.**60**). In both cases the patient's life expectancy of only a few months must be taken into consideration. For these patients it is therefore of even greater importance to regain as much of their natural laryngopharyngeal function as possible and thus maintain a better quality of life. The same guidelines that have been discussed for curative resections apply to the tumor ablation for palliative purposes.

> In comparison with curative operations, the risk of secondary hemorrhages is significantly higher after extensive palliative (tumor debulking) resections, especially if they extend far into the soft tissues of the neck.

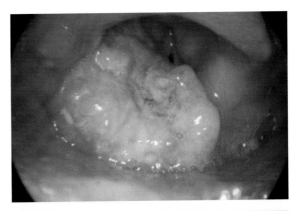

a

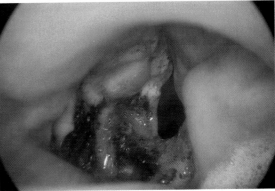

b

Fig. 3.**59**   This is an example of the limits of palliative transoral laser surgery. Patient A developed an obstruction from the recurrence of a hypoharynx carcinoma after radiotherapy. **a** Preoperative findings (endoscopic view, 90° telescope). **b** Postoperative situation as seen through the endoscope. The complete resection of the tumor was attempted at surgery. For this purpose large parts of the endolarynx had to be included in the resection. The resection reached onto the cricoid cartilage and large segments of the interarytenoid area were removed together with the left arytenoid cartilage. The patient suffered from severe aspiration postoperatively and had to undergo a tracheotomy. The tumor resection thus did not result in an improved quality of life for this patient. The difficulty of palliative and symptomatic tumor surgery lies in finding the balance between resecting as much as necessary and as little as possible to prevent severe functional disturbances in the postoperative period.

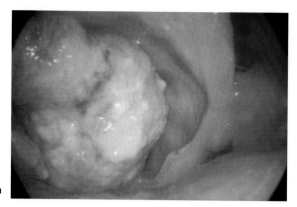

a

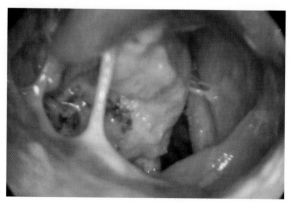

b

Fig. 3.**60**   This is an example of the opportunities offered by palliative-symptomatic transoral laser surgery. Patient B had an exophytically growing recurrence of a hypopharynx carcinoma after primary irradiation. This had caused symptoms of obstruction. **a** Preoperative situation (endoscopic view, 90° telescope). **b** Postoperative finding at endoscopy. A tracheotomy was avoided by performing a partial resection without a curative intent. This procedure obviously meant great relief for the patient. Undue radicality must be avoided in such palliative-symptomatic operations. The life expectancy of these patients averages between 6–9 months. Therefore, the laser surgery aims primarily at improving the quality of life, since a prolongation of the patient's life can usually not be achieved.

Laser Treatment for Malignant Tumors in Nose, Nasopharynx, and Trachea

Curative Microsurgery with the CO_2 Laser

In Europe malignant tumors of nose, nasopharynx, and trachea are rare compared to the squamous cell carcinomas of oral cavity, pharynx, and larynx. Primary tumors for which curative laser surgery can be considered are even less common. The endonasal, transoral, or translaryngeal route, which is chosen for minimally invasive surgery, does not always provide an adequate exposure in these narrow spaces. This is, however, an absolute prerequisite for the safe and complete resection of the tumor. We are of the opinion that the laser should be used as the cutting instrument for highly vascular tumors with a tendency for metastasis, regardless of the chosen access route.

The advantages of laser microsurgery, which have already been mentioned for the treatment of laryngeal and hypopharyngeal tumors, apply similarly to these cases. Briefly, these are the microscopic view, the bloodless field, and the sealing of lymphatic capillaries.

Tumors of the Nose and Paranasal Sinuses

Tumors can arise from the mucosal lining of the nose or paranasal sinuses, for example, septum, turbinates, or floor of nose. Small, circumscribed tumors that can be excised in one piece with an adequate resection margin are relatively rare in this area. It is, however, surprising what degree of precision can be maintained during the complete resection of lesions in the narrowest of spaces. It can be compared to laser treatment for choanal atresia in the newborn baby. Additional conventional electrocautery is usually required for resections in the area of the turbinates.

Our experience is, however, comparatively limited. We have treated more cases of obstruction from malignant lymphomas and melanomas with laser surgical methods than squamous cell carcinomas. A combined approach is recommended if the exposure is inadequate or in the case of tumors with particularly difficult access. The endonasal route is then combined with a lateral rhinotomy, or alternatively a midfacial degloving can be considered.

Tumors of the Nasopharynx

Cure has only rarely been the intention of our treatment of tumors in the nasopharynx. Apart from palliative treatment there are very few primary tumors in this area that are amenable to a microsurgical laser resection followed by radiotherapy and chemotherapy with curative intent. Infiltrating tumors, for example, with invasion of the skull base are a contraindication unless debulking of a very large, obstructing lesion is performed before radiochemotherapy. Depending on the exact localization and extent of the tumor, a temporary palatal split may become necessary. In some patients we have successfully removed the tumor with the laser via this transpalatal approach. These were cases of recurrence after irradiation that presented as superficial, more exophytic tumor growth.

Tumors of the Trachea

Squamous cell carcinomas are also rare in the trachea. It has been mentioned in the discussion of laryngeal carcinomas with subglottic extension that these tumors can be completely resected via a translaryngeal approach, even if there is tumor invasion into the proximal trachea. The prerequisites for these are good exposure and the absence of significant infiltration into the soft tissues of the neck.

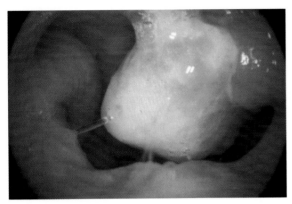
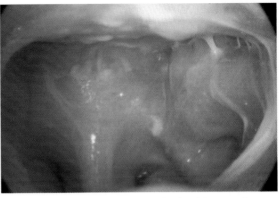

a

b

Fig. 3.**61** Recurrence of a nasopharynx carcinoma after radiotherapy. The documentation of findings before and after treatment with an argon laser is shown. **a** Preoperatively the exophytic tumor recurrence is seen in the right nasopharynx. **b** The findings after palliative argon laser ablation under endoscopic control.

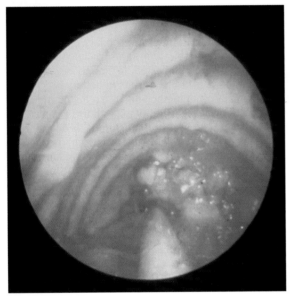
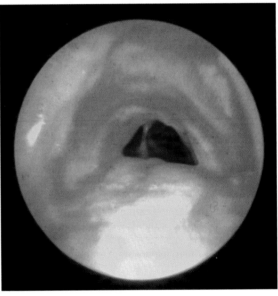

a

b

Fig. 3.**62** This is a case of an adenoidcystic carcinoma of the trachea with infiltration into the mediastinum. A palliative resection was performed with the argon laser and the preoperative and postoperative findings are documented. **a** An exophytic tumor can be recognized in the trachea. It has lead to an almost complete obliteration of the tracheal lumen. In the lower part of the photograph one can see the jet cannula which was used to ventilate the patient during the procedure. The operation was performed under endoscopic control with an argon laser. **b** The trachea after the palliative tumor resection. By carrying out this operation the patient was spared a tracheotomy.

If, however, the region of the tumor cannot be exposed adequately or in the case of a primary tracheal tumor, we use a combined approach. The trachea is split over the length of a few centimeters along the midline and explored under the microscope. The tumor is then resected according to its extent. Following the resection of superficially spreading squamous cell carcinomas or tumor recurrences, the trachea can be closed again primarily despite the resulting open wound surface within the tracheal lumen, which can be of quite substantial size. If cartilage has been extensively invaded with or without break-through into the soft tissues of the neck, the resection must be extended accordingly. In these cases we create an epithelialized, furrow-like tracheostoma, which is closed secondarily with a plastic-reconstructive technique after a recurrence-free interval of a few months.

Endoscopic or Microscopic Palliative Laser Treatment

Indications: Recurrences, metastases; malignant melanoma, adenoidcystic carcinoma, and others.

Type of laser: Argon, Nd:YAG, or CO_2 laser.

Application: Aided by rigid or flexible endoscopy.

The laser fiber is introduced under visual control either via a guiding device next to the rigid endoscope (paraendoscopic) or through a special instrument with integrated optics. The fiber can also be inserted through the instrument channel of flexible endoscopes.

At the beginning of the 1980s we mainly used the argon laser for palliative tumor treatment in nasopharynx and trachea (Fig. 3.**61** and 3.**62**). The tumor was vaporized in the process. More recently we have been using the CO_2 or Nd:YAG laser. The latter has the advantage of better coagulation during tumor resection by direct contact with the tissues. A disadvantage of the Nd:YAG laser is, however, the more pronounced heat generation spreading to the tissues surrounding the resection area. This can ultimately result in necrosis of neighboring structures, such as tracheal cartilage or the bones of the skull base.

The main difficulty with stenosing tumors of the trachea (Fig. 3.**62**) is the anesthetic management and especially the ventilation of the patient. Complications such as, for example, pneumothorax can occur if positive pressure ventilation such as jet ventilation is used. This is even more probable in cases with significant narrowing of the tracheal lumen by the space-occupying lesion. We prefer the application of the laser treatment in the apneic phase. An endotracheal tube is inserted intermittently through the laryngoscope and the patient ventilated under controlled circumstances during the treatment pauses. Disadvantages and difficulties encountered with this technique are mainly the lack of exposure, problems with smoke evacuation, and difficult control of larger hemorrhages.

We have performed a temporary tracheal split in some patients with very extensive tracheal stenoses from tumor masses. The tumor debulking was then performed with the CO_2 laser and a microsurgical technique from the external approach.

Perioperative Measures

Perioperative or Postoperative Tracheotomy vs. Intubation

In general we try to avoid a tracheotomy. An *indication* for a primary temporary tracheotomy is a very extensive partial resection of oropharynx, hypopharynx, and larynx with a high risk for secondary hemorrhages, for example, a patient on dialysis, severe liver cirrhosis with clotting abnormalities, or a high risk of aspiration.

Advantages of tracheotomy. The main advantage is the management of severe secondary bleeding. The cuff can be blocked immediately and a significant aspiration avoided. A pack can be inserted to control the bleeding without prior intubation. Another advantage is the possibility to start oral feeds earlier with a carefully inflated cuff. Patients with tracheal tube in situ aspirate less saliva, causing less irritation and coughing. This means less strain on the patient and a reduced risk of secondary hemorrhages.

The only indication for a secondary tracheotomy is persisting severe aspiration, although a permanent tracheotomy is rarely indicated. In these cases a speech valve can be used, which results in better speech function than any other method of voice rehabilitation after laryngectomy. If the inability to swallow is expected to last for several months or if the dysphagia does not improve as expected, a PEG tube should be inserted. A completion laryngectomy for functional reasons should be the last resort.

Delayed extubation. Immediate postoperative extubation is not recommended in all cases of very extensive partial resections of larynx and hypopharynx, especially in elderly patients. Extubation on the morning of the first postoperative day has been shown to be successful. When delayed extubation is decided upon, the patient is reintubated by the surgeon via the nose under direct vision at the end of the operation and admitted to an intensive care unit overnight. There are some advantages of this method: The patients have been awake for some time and are more cooperative. There is less immediate aspiration of saliva or secretions from the wound. Altogether the delayed extubation is better tolerated by patients, especially the elderly.

Medical Therapy

Neither antibiotics nor cortisone are generally necessary. The perioperative administration of antibiotics should be considered in cases of:
– large areas of exposed cartilage or bone,
– prolonged intubation for 24 hours.

The administration of cortisone is hardly ever necessary. It should only be given prophylactically if secondary edema is expected to form, leading to a possible airway obstruction.

Blood transfusions for intraoperative blood loss have so far not been necessary in our patients.

Postoperative Edema

Edema of the arytenoid area can develop if the resection line runs just superior to the arytenoid cartilage with preservation of the mucosa of the arytenoid and postcricoid area and simultaneous complete resection of the pyriform sinus. This edema rarely compromises the airway and hence does not require any treatment. The same applies for extensive partial resections of the larynx, where the arytenoid cartilage has been included in the resection but the pyriform sinus mucosa could be preserved.

If treatment is necessary, it is recommended to commence therapy by administering cortisone. If there is no improvement, the edema must be excised with the laser at microlaryngoscopy. The difficulty with this procedure is to resect as much as necessary to provide an adequate airway and as little as possible to prevent aspiration. The mucosal edema is difficult to visualize at microlaryngoscopy. There is a risk of removing too little if the mucosa is not held and retracted with a grasping forceps for adequate exposure.

Feeding Tube

The necessity for a feeding tube depends on the extent of the resection and the degree of the expected swallowing difficulties and aspiration. We do not routinely insert feeding tubes after the resection of early stages of tumors (T1 and small T2). If an extensive resection has been performed, we usually keep a thin nasogastric tube in place for a few days. The tube needs to stay in place for up to 1–2 weeks only if the arytenoid cartilage has been included in the resection. If an almost circumferential resection of the hypopharynx with possible inclusion of the esophageal inlet has been performed, we use one or two large-bore nasogastric feeding tubes. They are kept in for 3–4 weeks as stents due to the increased risk of scar formation leading to a stenosis.

Another reason for the insertion of a feeding tube is the risk of infection from food rests collecting in the wound cavity. If, for example, the entire pyriform sinus has been resected and large parts of the thyroid cartilage exposed in the process or removed, early oral feeding can result in the accumulation of food particles in the wound and eventually lead to an infection. An alternative is a fully liquid diet for a few days. As soon as the wound has started to form a protective layer of fibrin and granulation tissue over the cartilage, it is possible to change to a soft diet.

Wound Healing

The wound usually does not require any medical or surgical treatment at the end of the operation or in the postoperative period. An exception must be made if there is a risk of a secondary hemorrhage in patients where the transoral resection extended all the way into the neck. In these cases it is recommended to cover the wound from the inside with collagen mesh and fibrin glue.

The wounds heal *spontaneously*. A fibrinous layer forms and granulation tissue starts to form in the depth of the wound. The epithelization takes 1–4 weeks, depending on the size of the wound defect. Complete wound healing might even take a few months if cartilage or bone have been exposed during the resection of recurrent tumor after radiotherapy.

If an extensive resection of the pyriform sinus has been performed, including medial, anterior, and lateral walls, the wound surfaces can stick together, form fibrinous adhesions which cause a complete obliteration of the operated pyriform sinus by scar tissue. If the arytenoid cartilage has been preserved in the operation but the mucosa resected from its lateral aspect, it can be included in this scar. The individual response to the surgical wound will result in different degrees of lateral traction exerted on the arytenoid area after wound healing and scar formation have been completed. Reduced mobility and even the fixation of the arytenoid cartilage may result.

☞ Reduced mobility of the arytenoid cartilage in the postoperative period can be misinterpreted as submucosal tumor recurrence. This is one of the reasons why video documentation is so important. It is a valuable tool to help recognize reduced cord mobility developing slowly secondary to the formation of scar tissue as part of wound healing.

↯ There is strong suspicion of submucosal tumor recurrence if the arytenoid cartilage has been freely mobile for the first 2–3 months postoperatively and reduced mobility starts to develop after 5–6 months.

The differential diagnosis of persistent or worsening odynophagia in an irradiated patient includes tumor recurrence but also the infection or necrosis of cartilage. Imaging techniques (CT or MRI) and microlaryngoscopic examination help to solve this diagnostic dilemma. During the examination under the microscope, the scar tissue is carefully dissected and the underlying cartilage exposed. Biopsies are sent for histological assessment and will provide the answer as to whether it is an inflammatory, radiogenic reaction of the cartilage, or tumor recurrence.

The *fixation of the arytenoid cartilage from the surgical intervention* does not, however, have any significant functional repercussions, particularly no permanent swallowing problems. An impaired voice may result from an incomplete glottic closure. Some degree of fixation occurs almost always after the resection of tumors of the pyriform sinus with inferior extension and invasion of the medial wall (i.e., the lateral wall of the larynx). In early tumor stages or a lesser degree of involvement of the medial wall, the laryngeal function can usually be preserved entirely.

Intraoperative and Postoperative Hemorrhages—Prevention and Management

Preventive Measures to Reduce Blood Loss and Avoid Dangerous Bleeding

Preoperative Measures

Warfarin and aspirin must be stopped in time and clotting factors must be substituted in known cases of clotting abnormalities.

Tumor extension into the soft tissues of the neck can result in the encasing or infiltration of large vessels by tumor masses. In these cases and cases of vascular anomalies the topographical relationship between tumor and large vessels must be documented preoperatively by imaging techniques or angiography.

Intraoperative Measures

A special hypotensive anesthetic technique can be used. A head-down position should be avoided if at all possible. More severe hemorrhages *during the dissection* can be avoided by the following measures:

- Prophylactic electrocautery of feeding vessels for instance in the pharyngoepiglottic fold. The mucosa with the underlying feeding vessels is grasped laterally with the coagulation forceps and diathermized. The laser dissection can then proceed without bleeding. Dr Kim Davis (Salt Lake City – personal communication) recommends the prophylactic ligation of feeding vessels in the neck, including the external carotid artery for operations on hypopharyngeal carcinomas, when more severe intraoperative or postoperative bleeding is expected. So far we have found no reason to follow these guidelines routinely. In some cases of very extensive resections into the soft tissues of the neck we have, however, performed a prophylactic ligation of the external carotid artery. This was necessary because of very severe intraoperative bleeding or because of an exceptionally high risk of potentially fatal postoperative hemorrhages.
- Larger vessels can be better defined if the dissection is done carefully layer by layer and with low power settings. The suction diathermy cannula has proved especially useful as a dissecting instrument in these situations. Larger vessels can thus be identified earlier, before they are severed by the laser beam. They can then be controlled by conventional techniques with the suction diathermy or the coagulation forceps, depending on the localization and size of the vessel. This approach saves time and reduces the blood loss.

! During the dissection and in particular during the short pauses, the surgeon must watch out for pulsations of the lateral pharyngeal wall. The tissues should be repeatedly pushed medially by pressure from the outside with the fingers. As soon as one gets close to the larger vessels, one can usually see the vascular wall shine through the wound.

The power of the laser should be reduced the closer the operation gets to the vascular sheath in the neck. Conventional instruments should also be used for the delicate dissection. The suction cannula can be used to dissect and palpate; a small forceps may be useful to spread the tissues and define the layers. This is especially important if the tumor has grown into close proximity of the large blood vessels in the neck.

Under no circumstances should the suction diathermy be used for the purpose of coagulation. It is more advisable to employ the suction cannula as retractor of the tissues in the vicinity of the vessel. A coagulation forceps is introduced with the other hand and smaller to medium-sized vessels can then be carefully coagulated.

Intraoperative Hemostasis

The consistent and meticulous coagulation of blood vessels during the operation minimizes the risk of secondary hemorrhages and significantly reduces the intraoperative blood loss. In order to control the *bleeding from smaller vessels*, for example, in the area of the vocal cords it can be advantageous to compress the vessel with a small piece of gauze rather than use the suction cannula. The gauze can be soaked with epinephrine. If the bleeding cannot be controlled by these measures, the defocused laser beam can be used for coagulation purposes. Conventional and especially monopolar electrocautery with the suction diathermy or the coagulation forceps should rather be avoided in the area of the vocal cords. Damage to muscular and ligamentous structures is thereby prevented. In cases of more severe bleeding, a successful technique has been the use of swab and suction cannula simultaneously in order to first exactly localize the source of bleeding and then control it.

During the dissection, a smaller arterial vessel can be severed, resulting in a visible squirting hemorrhage. This might stop spontaneously as the vessel retracts during further dissection and gets compressed temporarily. This vessel must always be identified and coagulated, since if this is not done meticulously, there is a real danger of a secondary hemorrhage from the vascular stump that was left uncauterized.

Experience has shown that intraoperative coagulation with the suction diathermy held in the nondominant hand is quick and effective. Coagulation with the coagulating forceps can, however, be better aimed at the bleeding vessel and is therefore gentler to the surrounding tissues. The decision on which type of coagulation to use will depend largely on the individual situation. There is no doubt that the frequent conventional hemostasis is relatively time-consuming. During longer, more extensive, partial resections the continuous change of instruments can also be quite strenuous for the surgeon.

Control of smaller vessels far from large vessels. The coagulation is done carefully with the electrocautery set at low power. The suction cannula remains in the nondominant hand. After successful hemostasis, the laser operation can immediately be continued by controlling the micromanipulator with the dominant hand. If there is bleeding from the depth of the wound and the source cannot be identified, it is recommended to introduce a forceps with the one hand to retract tissue for a better exposure of the bleeding point and then coagulate with the suction cannula held in the other hand. A coagulation forceps can be used in place of the suction cannula, in which case the sucker is used to expose deeper-lying tissue layers and keep the operative field free of blood while the vessel is controlled with the forceps.

For the management of bleeding from medium-sized venous or arterial vessels the suction cannula should be held in the nondominant hand, while the dominant hand directs the coagulation forceps to grasp the blood vessel.

> External pressure applied by an assistant can be helpful in some cases of more severe bleeding. It helps to improve the exposure and can effect a temporary compression of the vessel.

The management of the hemorrhage requires some dexterity. A large sucker is manipulated with the one hand, while a swab is introduced with the other hand. If there is very strong bleeding, a second suction cannula can be introduced to suck up blood and to compress the gauze swab. The hemorrhage should be temporarily controlled or at least reduced with the suction diathermy. The tissue surrounding the larger vessel can then be carefully dissected either with conventional instruments or the laser in order to define the vessel and finally coagulate it safely with the forceps.

The introduction of vascular clips is only necessary for bleeding from *larger* and especially arterial vessels, for example, superior laryngeal artery, cricoid artery, and lingual artery. A *massive hemorrhage* is managed by packing and compressing the wound under simultaneous suctioning. The neck is subsequently opened from the outside and the feeding vessel ligated. If necessary, the external carotid artery is tied off in these cases. As previously described, the transcervical approach is routinely used for a simultaneous neck dissection.

Hemorrhages close to the vascular sheath. A forceps introduced with the nondominant hand is used to medially retract structures for a better exposure. The dominant hand manipulates a small suction cannula to dissect and define the vessel. Depending on the size of the vessel, the bleeding is controlled either with the curved coagulation forceps during retraction of the large vessels or a vascular clip is applied. At the end of the operation collagen mesh and fibrin glue are used to cover the large vessels in the depth of the wound. The patient remains intubated and is admitted overnight to an intensive care unit. A tracheotomy should be considered if there is an increased risk of a secondary hemorrhage. If the bleeding cannot be managed in this fashion, the neck must be opened to expose the large vessels and ligate the necessary branches.

Postoperative Hemorrhages

Secondary hemorrhages, especially of a more severe nature, are relatively rare, even after extensive resections leaving large wound surfaces that are left open for spontaneous healing. Also, the relatively frequently applied electrocautery of even larger vessels and early oral feeding do not seem to increase this risk. We have so far not lost any patients from a secondary hemorrhage after curative laser resection.

Management of Secondary Hemorrhage

- If there is little blood admixture to the saliva, the patient is observed and the wound examined tele-endoscopically. An operation is not necessary. Medical antihypertensive treatment might be considered if the blood pressure is high.
- If the patient repeatedly coughs up fresh, bright-red blood, they should be transferred to the intensive care unit and preparations be made for an emergency intubation or tracheotomy. The safest is the immediate exploration of the operated area, preferably under general anesthetic and endotracheal intubation.

Predilection sites for secondary hemorrhages. In the larynx the most commonly involved area is posterolateral, just anterior to the arytenoid cartilage. Other sites are above and lateral to the superior edge of the thyroid cartilage. In oropharynx and hypopharynx secondary bleeding occurs especially from the lateral wall.

It can be difficult to find the source of the bleeding due to the lowered blood pressure during the anesthesia, but also because of the retraction of the bleeding vessel into the soft tissues.

> It is, therefore, important to provoke bleeding by applying pressure from the outside and by manipulating the tissues from the inside with the suction cannula or other instruments. This will help identify the bleeding source.

It is important that the operation report contains detailed information on the intraoperative management of blood vessels and particularly on critical areas of excessively difficult hemostasis. The management of the bleeding again depends on the type and localization of the hemorrhage. It is decided intraoperatively whether electrocautery is sufficient, whether a clip must be applied, or a vessel like the external carotid artery ligated. Finally, a tracheotomy must be considered if there continues to be a high risk of bleeding.

Complications

In this section we report on complications that have occurred after transoral laser surgery at the Department of Otorhinolaryngology, University of Göttingen, Germany. The analysis comprises 704 tumor operations that were performed between August 1986 and December 1994. The 704 patients presented with previously untreated squamous cell carcinoma of all T-stages. The tumors were located in the oral cavity, oropharynx, hypopharynx, and larynx. The treatment was given with curative intent. There were 101 carcinomas of the oral cavity, 140 oropharyngeal tumors, and 98 hypopharyngeal lesions. The laryngeal tumors were divided into 280 glottic carcinomas and 85 supraglottic carcinomas.

Complications related to the technique. There were no complications from the use of the CO_2 laser, such as combustion of the endotracheal tube, skin burns, or injuries to the eyes.

Pulmonary and Cardiac Complications

Various pulmonary and cardiac complications were encountered in five patients (0.7%) on the basis of pre-existing diseases. Two patients developed a bacterial, another patient an atypical pneumonia. One patient required ventilation for 24 hours for respiratory failure of unclear cause. A further patient needed intensive care treatment for the control of left cardiac failure and finally there was one case of halothane-induced hepatitis.

Postoperative Hemorrhage

A secondary hemorrhage occurred in the postoperative phase in 22 cases from a total of 704 intraoral or transoral tumor resections (3.1% of cases). Following the resection of carcinomas of the oral cavity, a secondary hemorrhage was seen in 3.9% of cases (4 out of 101 operations); three of the patients had early stages and one an advanced stage of disease. After resections for oropharyngeal carcinomas, there was postoperative bleeding in 6.4% of cases (9 out of 140 operations; three for early tumor stages, six for advanced cancers). It is interesting to look at the propensity of the different subsites of the oropharynx for the development of secondary hemorrhages after a resection. We experienced seven cases of secondary bleeding after the resection of tonsil carcinomas (7 out of 72 resections; 9.7%) and two subsequent to resections of vallecula tumors. Secondary hemorrhages occurred in 3.0% of resections of hypopharynx tumors (3 out of 98 operations), all of them early tumor stages. No postoperative bleeding was observed in any of the 280 patients with glottic carcinomas, but in 7.0% of partial supraglottic resections (6 out of 85 operations; three after surgery for early and three for advanced tumor stages).

In 19 cases electrocautery was used to control the bleeding under general anesthetic and endotracheal intubation. In three cases the bleeding was so severe that the external carotid artery had to be ligated from a transcervical approach and blood transfusion became necessary (maximum of three units). In the other 19 cases the bleeding had no significant influence on the hemoglobin concentration. There was no case of aspiration of blood that required treatment. One patient, who had a secondary hemorrhage after an extensive partial resection of the supraglottis, needed a tracheotomy due to intubation difficulties.

Eighty-two percent of the secondary hemorrhages occurred within the first 7 postoperative days. During the surgical management of these cases, the most common finding was that of a vessel that had reopened after having been coagulated during the initial surgery. The more frequent use of vascular clips leads to greater safety of controlling the bleeding vessel. This might lower the rate of secondary hemorrhages after resections of both oropharyngeal and supraglottic carcinomas. During the second postoperative week only mild bleeding occurred, mainly from the granulation tissue that had already formed in the wound at that stage.

All patients were still in hospital when the complication occurred. It is our opinion that patients who had more extensive resections, particularly in the oropharynx and the supraglottis, must be kept in hospital for at least 1 week after the operation. This makes immediate intervention possible in the case of a secondary hemorrhage. It is even more important if no prophylactic tracheotomy had been performed.

There was one patient who had a supraglottic, partial laryngectomy for a pT2 lesion supraglottic carcinoma. A secondary hemorrhage occurred on the day of the operation but could be controlled at microlaryngoscopy. The patient died the following day and a postmortem examination could not identify the cause of death. There were, however, definitely no signs of another hemorrhage.

Postoperative Mucosal Edema

In our entire patient population there were only four patients who required a tracheotomy either because of the primary tumor or as part of the surgery for the primary tumor.

Three patients were treated with high doses of glucocorticosteroids for several days for postoperative mucosal edema that had developed after an extensive transoral partial laryngectomy. In two additional patients mucosal edema that had lead to a compromise of the airway was surgically ablated with the CO_2 laser at microlaryngoscopy. One of these patients had a resection of a hypopharyngeal carcinoma and subsequently developed edema of the mucosa of the aryepiglottic fold, which prolapsed into the endolarynx. It was removed with the laser. The other patient developed edema in the area of the arytenoid cartilages subsequent to an extended partial resection of the supraglottis and postoperative irradiation treatment. This condition required repeated treatment with the laser.

Surgical Emphysema

Occasionally after resection of carcinomas of the anterior commissure and the subglottis, surgical emphysema has developed following penetration of the cricothyroid ligament. Surgical emphysema may then extend to involve the face and chest. This complication occurs when there is a surgical defect in the area of the cricothyroid ligament in a patient with normal function of the arytenoid cartilages and hence the ability to achieve full glottic closure. Subglottic pressure can build up and result in the extraluminal spread of air. In spite of extensive swelling, a tracheostomy has never been necessary. After more extensive operations, there is usually some form of glottic incompetence in the immediate postoperative period so that pressure cannot built up subglottically, and surgical emphysema is rare. When circumstances may increase the risk of emphysema, manual pressure or a compression bandage should be used during extubation when laryngeal spasm may lead to high subglottic pressure and extravasation of air.

Infection

In one insulin-dependent diabetic patient an abscess developed in the right pyriform sinus 3 months after resection of a pT1 hypopharynx carcinoma. This patient did not have any postoperative radiotherapy. The abscess was drained endoscopically and at the same time the necrotic remnants of the right arytenoid cartilage and some granulation tissue were removed. The patient received antibiotics and made an unremarkable recovery. Most importantly, no chondritis or osteomyelitis developed in the thyroid cartilage. Perichondritis and cartilaginous sequestra have occurred rarely, and in our experience, is associated with resecting recurrences after radiation.

Stenosis and Web Formation

Two female patients developed a supraglottic stenosis of the larynx after laser surgical resection of parts of the supraglottis. The stenosis in one of the patients could be managed by two endoscopic procedures without a tracheotomy. The other patient, who had preoperative bilateral recurrent nerve palsy from thyroid surgery, required a tracheotomy. In another patient extensive scarring of the anterior glottis and subglottis necessitated a tracheotomy. He had undergone a transoral laser resection for a bilateral glottic carcinoma with extensive subglottic spread (pT2). The patient refused any further surgery to resect the web.

Some patients, after extensive and repeated surgery for local recurrences, have developed stenosis in the cricoid area. This has been more marked after radiation therapy. Some of these patients have been subjected to reconstruction of the cricoid ring by interposition of rib cartilage and other techniques.

The formation of stenosis has been rare after laser surgery of either glottic or supraglottic carcinomas. This may be due to the fact that there is no loss of cartilage, as the cartilaginous skeleton is usually fully preserved during the laser procedure. Secondly, the development of clinically apparent chondritis is very rare. Finally, a maximum of healthy mucosa is preserved during the surgery.

Swallowing Problems

Three patients needed a temporary tracheotomy for aspiration after extended supraglottic partial resections (3/4 laryngectomy and partial pharyngectomy). A total laryngectomy had to be performed in one patient due to severe aspiration. The patient had an extensive partial resection of the supraglottis for a pT4 supraglottic carcinoma with invasion of the oropharynx and spread to both vocal folds. The histological examination of the larynx specimen showed no tumor.

Some degree of aspiration is a well-known phenomenon in many patients after more extensive vertical and particularly horizontal partial laryngectomies. The incidence of aspiration and of secondary pulmonary complications depends on the extent of the resection and the inclusion of functionally important structures such as arytenoid cartilage and tongue base. Paralysis of the laryngeal nerves and the pharyngeal branches of the vagus or the hypoglossal nerve can also be an important factor in the development of postoperative aspiration beside the resection of an arytenoid cartilage and parts of the tongue base. There are always nerves damaged during a classical vertical or horizontal partial laryngectomy. This nerve injury can add to the problem of postoperative aspiration due to decreased endolaryngeal and pharyngeal sensation or impaired muscle function. During transoral laser surgery, both recurrent nerves and the external branches of the superior laryngeal nerves can usually be spared. This is probably the reason for the improved preservation of sensation.

Summary

Comparisons with studies from the literature reveal that complications in the postoperative phase are not more common in our group of patients after intraoral or transoral partial laser resection of carcinomas of the upper aerodigestive tract than they are in patients who undergo a classical operation. All the complications that did arise could be managed.

If the airway is not secured with a tracheotomy, meticulous hemostasis and an atraumatic surgical technique are required to avoid secondary hemorrhages and the formation of postoperative edema. Clinically apparent infections are rare and fistula formation and its sequelae do not occur for reasons inherent to the method.

Microsurgery with the laser allows the exact adjustment of the resection to the extension of the tumor. In the process, structures that are important for voice and swallowing functions are more carefully preserved. In addition this prevents the development of stenoses and severe glottic incompetence and lays the basis for an improved postoperative rehabilitation of the swallowing function.

Aftercare

The purpose of oncological aftercare is the early detection of local recurrences, metastases, and second primary tumors. Laser microsurgery of tumors of the upper aerodigestive tract creates excellent conditions for an effective tumor aftercare. There are a number of simple investigations that can be performed in the outpatient department and that are well tolerated by the patients. These include tele-endoscopy, smear and fine needle aspiration cytology, palpation, and B-scan ultrasound examination of the area of the primary tumor and the neck. Routine microlaryngoscopy under general anesthesia is usually not necessary if these methods are used.

☞ Routine examination with CT or MRI is not required. Exceptions to this can be made after the resection of, for example, tumors of the base of tongue or subglottic carcinomas. However, if there is suspicion of a larger recurrence, these imaging modalities are indispensable for the diagnosis and evaluation of operability.

Documentation of the local findings in the form of photos or videos offer the opportunity for comparison as part of the follow-up of the patient after completion of the treatment. If no photographic equipment is available, the documentation of the findings in the form of sketches can be very helpful. In all cases the findings should be routinely and systematically documented in writing.

It is, for instance, advisable to always record the condition of the mucosa, the presence of granulation tissue, hyperplasia, scar tissue, or smooth prominences (which might hint at a submucosally growing tumor recurrence). Following a partial resection of larynx or hypopharynx, the mobility of the vocal cords should also always be documented.

The follow-up examinations should be performed at the treating center and preferably by the surgeons themselves, as they are the ones who have the most intricate knowledge of a particular patient and their problems. This enables them to put postoperative findings such as, for example, formation of granulation or scar tissue into the right perspective.

At most institutions tumor aftercare follows a rigid schedule. In our experience it is better to *individualize* the time schedule and adjust it to the particular patient. When the intervals of the follow-up visits are determined, prognostic factors should be considered, such as localization of the primary tumor, UICC/AJCC stage of the disease, resection margins (clear or narrow margins), and individual risk factors. A patient in whom an early glottic carcinoma was resected with a wide margin does not need to be followed up in 4-weekly intervals. In such a case examinations at intervals of 3–4 months are perfectly adequate. On the other hand, a patient who had no treatment of an N0 neck with high risk for clinically occult micrometastases must definitely be followed up in 4-8 weekly intervals during the final two years.

When the aftercare schedule is planned, it must also be considered whether the possibility of curative therapy still exists in the case of a *recurrence*. Further organ-sparing surgery is usually still possible for smaller, well-circumscribed recurrences that are detected early if the tumor had been primarily treated with an organ-sparing partial resection and curative intent. This is especially true for the larynx, where a tumor recurrence can often be treated by further partial resections and almost always by a total laryngectomy aiming at cure for the patient.

During the first 2 years after the treatment, the *regional lymph drainage* area should be examined sonographically at regular intervals for the early identification of late or recurrent metastases. If the neck disease is limited to smaller lymph nodes, an operation can still have a good chance of success, especially if no radiotherapy was given during the initial therapy. The chances of repeated treatment are significantly worse in cases of advanced recurrent cervical metastases, particularly if adjuvant irradiation treatment had been given. Often only palliative procedures are possible in these patients.

The problem of *distant metastases* underlines the discrepancy between diagnostic efficacy and resulting therapeutic implications. Regular chest radiographs and sonographic examinations of the liver are of dubious value as screening tests for distant metastases. An early detection is barely possible with these investigations. In addition, the lung and liver metastases of head and neck tumors are usually multiple and are only treated once they become symptomatic.

An important aspect of tumor aftercare is the early detection of *second primary tumors* in the upper aerodigestive tract and in the bronchi. Approximately one in five patients will develop a metachronous second primary. Tumor patients with a high risk of multiple tumors should therefore be examined regularly, so that at least some of the tumors in the head and neck region are detected at an early stage, when they are still curable. The examination can be restricted to routine tele-endoscopy under topical anesthesia. Endoscopic examination of the upper esophagus and bronchi under general anesthesia should only be performed if there are any symptoms.

Oncologically effective aftercare and sound psychological support for the patient require effective cooperation between general practitioner, private otorhinolaryngologist in the patient's home town, treatment center, and rehabilitation center. These are the prerequisites for optimal patient care and the best possible quality of life for the cancer patient.

4 Anesthesiological Aspects of Laser Surgery in Otorhinolaryngology

Minimally invasive laser surgery in the upper aerodigestive tract relies on precise cuts performed within the narrowest of spaces. It has brought a problem to the foreground that has not featured in the mind of anesthesiologists since the times of ether anesthesia, namely the danger of fires and explosion. The laser beam produces high temperatures at the spot where it is incident on tissue or other materials, with the potential to cause flammable materials to ignite (Chapter 6, p. ■ ff.). The main concern of the anesthesiological aspect of laser surgery is, therefore, the prevention of potentially life-threatening complications such as combustion or explosions by prophylactic measures.

Apart from the preventive steps, the anesthesiologist as well as the surgeon should have detailed knowledge of the measures and the correct order that are necessary in case of such a complication. The shared airway is the same inherent problem in laser surgery of the upper aerodigestive tract as it is for other operative procedures in this area. This means that surgical and anesthesiological tasks both have to be carried out within a very small space. Obviously, mutual understanding in general and specific planning of the individual treatment is necessary for a successful and safe operation. In addition to these topics, some special aspects of the intraoperative and postoperative phase of otorhinolaryngological laser surgery will be discussed.

The CO_2 laser is the most important instrument for the treatment of benign and malignant neoplasms in oropharynx, hypopharynx, and larynx. Its advantages are the limited depth of penetration into tissue and a cutting technique which is exact and easily controlled. The Nd:YAG laser can be used via optic fibers and is more commonly employed in trachea and bronchial tree. Due to its capacity for deeper penetration it can, however, result in greater tissue damage and therefore a higher complication rate. It is mainly used to alleviate airway obstruction from tumor masses in trachea and bronchi without the quest for operative radicality.

The impartiality of laser applications in the pioneering days of laser surgery in the 1970s and 1980s resulted in complications such as swabs catching fire, endotracheal tube and cuff explosions, burns of airway and lung parenchyma, as well as burns of face, lips, and eyes (Mayne et al., 1991; Ossoff, 1989; Padfield and Stamp, 1992; Wolf and Simpson, 1987). Fortunately, persisting defects were almost never reported. During the detailed investigation of these incidents the hazardous factors were identified. This resulted in a number of general and discipline-specific recommendations being made.

Fire Hazards

The prerequisites for an intraoperative fire or explosion are ignition or the necessary temperatures, flammable material, and an atmosphere that can sustain a fire.

The temperatures effected by the laser in tissue range from 60 °C for thermal denaturation of tumor tissue to 80–100 °C for the coagulation of blood vessels and 100–250 °C for the vaporization of tissue (see Chapter 6, p. ■ ff.). The very high temperatures result in dry, carbonized tissue. Small tissue particles or other materials can then combust locally in the focus of the laser. A temperature of more than 1000° can thereby develop in a small area and this is certainly enough to ignite any flammable substance. The further course depends on the amount of combustible material and the gas composition and supply.

Dry swabs, endotracheal tube materials, and even an adequate amount of carbonized tissue can feature as flammable material. Several different tube materials, such as red rubber, silicone, and polyvinyl chloride (PVC), have been tested with regards to their combustibility (Wolf and Simpson, 1987). Combustibility was defined as the ability to maintain a flame in a defined environment. After a defined ignition, rubber burned at an oxygen concentration of 17.6 %, silicone at 18.9 %, and PVC at 26.3 % (Table 4.**1**). This means that PVC is the least flammable under these conditions, although toxic hydrocarbons are released during its combustion, including substances such as methylchloride, ethylchloride, propylchloride, vinylchloride, as well as substantial quantities of hydrochloric acid (Foth et al., 1991). Silicone is relatively easily flammable, it scorches at low laser power and oxidizes to silicone dioxide, the white silica ash residue. This inorganic substance interferes with wound healing, can cause formation of granulation tissue, and may present a long-term hazard from silicosis. Red rubber burns more slowly, its smoke is less toxic to the lung parenchyma, and it does not leave harmful residues.

☞ Rubber, silicone, and PVC are not suited as materials for endotracheal tubes used in laser surgery.

Effect of the Inspired Anesthetic Gasses on Combustion

The gas inspired by the patient during a general anesthesia contains oxygen, nitrous oxide or nitrogen, and the volatile anesthetics. Helium can be used under special operative circumstances.

Oxygen. The ability of the oxygen molecule to take up electrons during the oxidative process explains the role that it has in cell respiration and the process of combustion. Ignition and burning of a substance are dependent on the presence of oxygen. Any increase in the oxygen concentration above the atmospheric partial pressure leads to an increase in reactivity. For all practical purposes of laser surgery, a compromise is recommended with an oxygen concentration of 30 %.

☝ During laser surgery only use 30 % oxygen concentration!

Nitrous oxide (N$_2$O). Nitrous oxide is stable under the normal thermal conditions of the human body. The molecule disintegrates at a temperature of 300 °C or more and is then able to sustain a fire (Merck & Co., 1976; Mushin and Jones, 1987; Wolf and Simpson, 1987). This is the reason why nitrous oxide is used as an oxidant for organic substances and as a component of rocket fuel. It complements the ability of oxygen to sustain a fire (Wolf and Simpson, 1987). Therefore, the recommendation has been made to avoid this anesthetic gas on principle during laser surgical procedures.

⚡ No nitrous oxide during laser operations!

Air. Room air can be used for anesthesiological purposes since many anesthetic machines have circuits that allow the addition of room air to the employed gas mixture. In the old anesthetic machine Engstroem 300, room air is added via a Venturi gas mixing apparatus. The Spiromat 656 by Dräger, Germany, has a separate compressed air line installed on the machine. The Sulla 19 by the same company and other older machines only have the options of oxygen and nitrous oxide. They are thus not suitable for laser surgery, since only pure oxygen can be used if nitrous oxide is avoided. A modification of these older machines by the manufacturer is a possibility. This, however, requires the approval according to federal governmental regulations. If there is the option for room air supplementation of the anesthetic gas as in the Dräger Cato, a low flow of fresh oxygen is sufficient to achieve a concentration of 30 % in the inspiratory gas mixture.

☝ The nitrogen in the air dampens the reactivity of chemical interactions leading to combustion, decreases the combustibility of substances, and reduces the amount of thermal energy produced.

Table 4.**1** Flammability and burn residues of different materials used for endotracheal tubes

Material used for tube	Oxygen concentration required for combustion (%)	Burn residues
Red rubber	17.8	–
Silicone	18.9	White silica ash
PVC	26.3	Toxic hydrocarbons, Hydrochloric acid

Helium. Helium is superior to nitrogen in its ability to quench the process of combustion (Ossoff, 1989). Its physical properties also make it a helpful adjunct in cases of difficult ventilation. On the other hand, the use of helium has great logistic and financial implications which obviate its routine use. After all, the use of air together with all the measures of fire and explosion prevention provide sufficient safety and security.

Volatile anesthetics. The commonly used volatile anesthetics are halothane, enflurane, isoflurane, desflurane and sevoflurane. Their combination with air is not flammable under normal clinical circumstances (Merck & Co., 1986). Combustibility is theoretically possible at concentrations of nine times the MAC (minimal alveolar concentration) factor (enflurane 9 MAC, isoflurane 15 MAC, halothane 17 MAC). The MAC value is a pharmacological measure for the depth of the anesthesia and the tolerance toward a standardized surgical stimulus. At an alveolar concentration of approximately 0.8 % halothane, 50 % of anesthetized patients do not show any reaction to the applied standardized pain stimulus (1 MAC).

General Guidelines for Patient Safety

The eyes of the patient should be protected by special eye shields or covered with swabs soaked in saline. We use a thin stripe of plaster to keep the eyes closed. Skin protection is also effectively achieved with wet towels, as the CO$_2$ laser radiation is absorbed by water. Also, the mucosal surface in the immediate proximity of the operative field should be protected by moistened swabs. The protective swabs and towels should be wetted at regular intervals during the procedure.

Special mention must be made of the protective eyeglasses used for argon lasers. Their use results in a significant impairment of the assessment of the patient's skin color. As the anesthetist will also be required to wear these shields, a serious situation could arise as a decrease in the oxygen saturation of the patient might be missed. Adequate monitoring devices are mandatory (see p. 120ff).

Choice of Anesthetic

Continuous intravenous anesthetic techniques are basically suited for laser surgery, as is inhalation anesthesia. The decision for the one or the other technique is among other factors dependent on the question of whether the patient is intubated endotracheally or whether the ventilation is maintained otherwise. The choice of the individual anesthetic agent depends on personal preferences and experiences, but also on the pharmacological properties of the particular substance.

Among the intravenous combinations of drugs we have had particularly good experiences with propofol together with alfentanil or remifentanil. The dosage for continuous intravenous administration is 4-10 mg/kg/h for propofol with a dose reduction during the course of a longer operation. Alfentanil is administered at 0.3–0.6 µg/kg/min and remifentanil at 0.2–0.4 µg/kg/min.

These drugs are well tolerated by the patient and allow for good control over the general anesthetic. They are also indicated in short procedures, when the drug can be administered by hand. Furthermore, propofol reduces the activity of reflexes in the area of pharynx and larynx. Bradycardia, which is a possible side effect of propofol, can be dealt with by prophylactic administration of the anticholinergic glycopyrrolate (Robinul). For longer procedures the combination of midazolam with fentanyl or sufentanil is more advisable, although the use of propofol with ketamine or midazolam with ketamine is also a possibility.

Halothane and isoflurane can be employed; their use, however, should be restricted to endotracheal intubation in a cuffed system. Otherwise, inadmissible contamination of the environment may occur. The volatile anesthetics can only be used without nitrous oxide and must therefore be administered in doses higher than those used in combination with this anesthetic gas. The use of an opioid decreases the required dose of the volatile anesthetic. Combinations with alfentanil, remifentanil, fentanyl, or sufentanil in the form of a balanced anesthesia might be considered.

Induction of Anesthesia

The details of the induction depend on the type of procedure planned, on the condition of the airway with special reference to the patient's disease, and the experience of the anesthesiologist. Apart from the particulars of the intubation, most other steps and measures are not dictated by the laser surgical treatment.

In cases of airway obstruction from bulky laryngeal carcinomas the patient is first ventilated with a mask. After the administration of a muscle relaxant a 25° telescope is introduced through a semi-closed laryngoscope and the larynx and trachea are inspected. Then the intubation follows under visual control. If a difficult intubation is anticipated, fiber optic intubation in the awake patient is the first choice. If a feeding tube is required due to the anticipation of swallowing problems postoperatively, this should not be inserted during the induction of the anesthetic but under visual guidance after the surgical treatment has been completed. This also has the advantage that no further flammable material is introduced into the surgical field.

Muscle Relaxants

Muscle relaxation is not generally required for laser surgical procedures except for intubation, introduction of the operating laryngoscope, jet ventilation, and ventilation through the bronchoscope. A deep anesthetic and good analgesia are further requirements for the insertion of the operating laryngoscope. Among the available muscle relaxants, rocuronium, cisatracurium, atracurium, vecuronium, and pancuronium are suitable.

Scoline has a long list of side effects, such as cardiac arrhythmias, release of potassium, and histamine release with allergic reaction. The medium-long acting substances such as atracurium and vercuronium and more recently rocuronium and cisatracurium have to some extent replaced scoline. Muscle relaxants, especially the medium-long acting drugs, are today commonly given through continuous intravenous administration. Methods of assessing the degree of relaxation, such as nerve stimulators, should be used routinely.

We prefer the use of rocuronium today because of its short response time.

Rocuronium, atracurium, cisatracurium, or vecuronium should be used for muscle relaxation.

Endotracheal Intubation

An endotracheal tube is the safest method of securing an airway and offers a great degree of protection against aspiration. The volatile anesthetic gases and oxygen are kept out of the operative field and optimal monitoring of ventilation and gas concentration is made possible. The disadvantage lies in the occupation of space in the immediate vicinity of the surgical field. We try to perform the operations under endotracheal intubation whenever this is technically possible. Occasionally, it becomes necessary to change the position of the tube during the course of the operation, as the laser beam must be used from a different angle to continue the procedure. The temporary removal of the tube after adequate oxygenation of the patient (apnoe technique) is a further possibility to allow laser treatment to areas with difficult access, particularly in the region of the posterior larynx or the trachea.

The first reports on surgical applications of the laser make mention of two weak points (Padfield and Stamp, 1992; Perera and Mallon, 1987; Sosis and Dillon, 1991). The one is the use of red rubber as material for endotracheal tubes, the other the cuff which was filled with air or—via diffusion—with nitrous oxide. The cuff is inevitably situated in the path of the laser radiation.

In those days the problem was solved wrapping metal foil around the endotracheal tube. In the meantime it has been shown that this does not provide adequate protection and actually produces additional hazards. The foils can come loose and cause airway obstruction as well as injuries to the mucosa.

The cuff problem was solved by filling it with 0.9 % saline solution, which made sure that a cuff explosion became impossible (Fig. 4.1). It must be remembered that both filling and emptying of the cuff with saline require significantly more time than air. If the saline-inflated cuff is exposed to the laser beam, it is destroyed. A reintubation is then unavoidable, which is the only disadvantage.

Three solutions to the tube problem can be recommended with today's standards of quality control. They differ significantly in concept and price (Table 4.2,

Table **4.2** Some characteristics of four endotracheal tubes. An inner diameter (ID) of 6 mm has been used as standard for the comparison. **1** MLT: special ENT tube by Mallinckrodt (microlaryngeal tube). **2** MLT + LG: Merocel laser guard by Rüscher, Pattensen, Germany. **3** Laser-Trach by Sheridan. **4** Laser shield II: Xomed Treace. **5** Laser flex: metal tube by Mallinckrodt.

	MLT[1]	MLT + LG[2]	Laser Shield II[3]	Laser Trach[4]	Laser Flex[4]
Material	PVC	Corrugated silver foam layer containing water	Silicone + double layer of aluminium and teflon	Fabric-covered, embossed copper foil-wrapped red rubber	Metal
Outer diameter (mm) for ID 6 mm	8.0	11.0	9.0	10.6	8.5
Wall Thickness	1.0	2.5	1.5	2.3	1.25
Time until combustion occurs, for direct continuous irradiance with 35 watt	2 seconds	> 3 minutes	> 3 minutes	> 3 minutes	> 3 minutes
Advantage	Space saving	Laserproof	Laserproof	Laserproof	Laserproof
Disadvantage	Unprotected	Space occupying		Space occupying	
Special features		Tube difficult to distinguish from tissue	Methylene blue cristals within the cuff	Tube difficult to distinguish from tissue	Double cuff
Company	Mallinckrodt	Mallinckrodt Xomed-Treace	Xomed-Treace	Sheridan	Mallinckrodt

Fig. **4.2**). The cheapest solution is the well-tried MLT tube made from PVC combined with a laser-proof cover consisting of corrugated silver foil and sponge soaked in water (Merocel laser guard). The double protection through metal foil and water even resists direct radiation with the laser for several minutes (Foth et al., 1991). The significant additional thickness defies the favorable ratio of inner to outer diameter, which is an advantage of the MLT tube. This can lead to practical problems during laser procedures in very narrow spaces such as the larynx. Either surgeons perform the operation without the protective cover and places wet swabs to shield tube and cuff, or they primarily opt for the insertion of a different endotracheal tube (see below). Another practical problem with the Merocel laser guard is the discoloration of the sponge. The material stains red from the admixture of blood to the watery solution used to soak it. This can make it difficult to distinguish the cuff from the surrounding tissues. In general, an endotracheal tube is used with an inner diameter of 6 mm. In most cases this guarantees a safe anesthetic management. The combination of MLT tube and Merocel laser guard is a useful and cost-effective solution which is indicated especially for operations in the area of oral cavity and pharynx. The layer of Merocel laser guard should be applied to the tube at least 30 minutes before it is used. After the application of the protection, the tube is placed in a solution of 0.9 % saline to fully saturate the merocel layer.

We also use the MLT tube without the protective cover in order to save space if the operation takes place under conditions of very limited access due to anatomical circumstances.

It is important to pay attention to the tube during the operation and protect it with wet swabs where necessary. The accidental tangential incidence of the laser beam on the tube does not cause any damage.

Our experience with this tube has been good. However, we cannot generally recommend the above-mentioned practice for reasons of inadequate laser safety.

Our own experiments showed that the wall of this endotracheal tube is perforated after continuous direct irradiance with the laser for 30 seconds at 5 W, after 11 seconds at 10 W, and after 2 seconds at 35 W. The tube is quite resistant to laser radiation with a tangentially incident beam and a power setting of 5 W, as is commonly used in clinical practice.

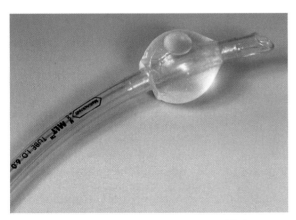

Fig. **4.1** The MLT tube by Mallinckrodt, is suitable for microlaryngeal operations. It is shown with the cuff filled with saline.

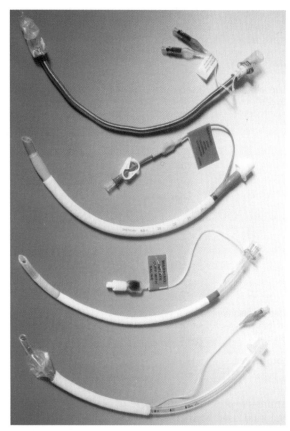

Fig. 4.**2**   Four endotracheal tubes suited for laser surgery. From bottom to top: MLT tube by Mallinckrodt, with the Merocel laser guard cover; Laser shield II tube by Xomed-Treace; Sheridan Laser Trach; Laser flex tube by Mallinckrodt (see text for details).

Another very suitable tube is the Laser shield II by Xomed-Treace. This is the successor of the Laser shield I, which was manufactured from silicone with a superficial metal coating. Subsequent to an intra-operative combustion of the cuff, this predecessor was taken off the market (Blomquist et al., 1990). The new development is characterized by a double coating of a silicone tube with aluminum and Teflon without the use of an adhesive. The cuff is protected by small cloth pieces which come with the tube and only need to be moistened. The connector for the inflation of the cuff contains methylene blue crystals. These will stain the saline solution in the cuff and facilitate the detection of an intraoperative cuff leak. The cuff withstands direct, continuous laser radiation at 35 W or more for 3 minutes.

The Laser Trach tracheal tube is a fabric covered, embossed copper foil-wrapped red rubber tube, which is resistent to carbon dioxide, but not to Nd-YAG laser radiation.

The Laser flex tube by Mallinckrodt, Germany, has been found to be the safest endotracheal tube by several investigators (Hawkins and Joseph, 1990; Padfield and Stamp, 1992; Werner et al., 1990). This is a spiral tube of metal which fulfills many of the requirements of laser surgery. It resists the direct irradiance with high powers for longer than any other tube, and the danger of perforation or explosion is practically nonexistent under clinical circumstances. This tube has two cuffs, the proximal of which protects the distal against the laser beam. A disadvantage is the great scattering effect on the radiation and reflective properties of the Laser flex. This can, in principle, lead to tissue damage. Apart from this, it is slightly stiff in the handling.

Laryngeal Mask Airway (LMA)

The LMA which has been devised by Brain is an almost noninvasive means to secure the airway. Its concept and function is placed somewhere between the endotracheal tube and the face mask (Braun and Fritz, 1994; White, 1991). It adapts to the pharynx like an air cushion (Fig. 4.**3**). The technique of introduction is easier than endotracheal intubation. The method is very safe for ENT interventions, but does not constitute a reliable protection against aspiration. The correct patient selection is of crucial importance to avoid this problem. The LMA allows a very smooth wake-up phase and no muscle relaxants are necessary for its use. It can also be used as an instrument to gain access to the exposed larynx and the trachea. This is, for instance, of importance for its use in conjunction with the Nd:YAG laser, which is employed for palliative reopening of the airway in cases of partial obstruction of trachea or bronchial tree. This laser is applied via a flexible bronchoscope which is introduced through the laryngeal mask. The advantage of this technique is the absence of any instrumentation in the airway distal to the larynx. Another favorable circumstance is the inner diameter of the connecting tube of the laryngeal mask, which has a larger lumen than that of an endotracheal tube and thus provides more operative space. A slight disadvantage is the free distribution of the laser plume within the airways. It must, however, be borne in mind that these operations on trachea and bronchi are usually short procedures, with very acute indications. They are often performed as emergency operations to avoid acute asphyxiation of the patient.

Monitoring

The most important instruments for the clinical monitoring are eye, ear, hand, and possibly nose of the anesthesiologist, who should be specially trained in clinical observation. There are no differences between the monitoring for an anesthetic using an endotracheal tube or an LMA. Optimal monitoring is possible for both methods of airway control and together with the clinical observation a safe general anesthesia can be guaranteed. The method of minimal monitoring is usually adequate (Braun and Fritz, 1994). This includes electrocardiogram (ECG) monitor with pulse rate display, body temperature, as well as tidal volume and ventilating pressures if the patient is connected to a ventilator. The anesthetic ventilation is monitored by controlling the inspiratory oxygen concentration, the use of alarms to indicate disconnection, stenosis, fall of oxygen concentration, and a nitrous oxide gate.

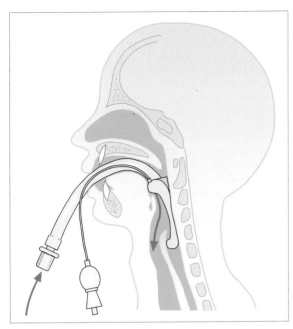

Fig. 4.**3**   Schematics of the laryngeal mask in situ. The device adjusts to the pharyngeal entrance without touching the larynx.

In Germany the monitoring and control of ventilation is automatically in accordance with the requirements of federal regulation for medical devices. In keeping with the developments of recent years the noninvasive techniques of capnometry and pulse oxymetry should be included in the range of minimal monitoring. More invasive monitoring such as central venous or intra-arterial pressure reading is rarely necessary for laser surgical procedures. These measures might, however, be indicated for patients with significant systemic disease and for prolonged operations. A urinary catheter should be inserted when the duration of the operation definitely exceeds 2–3 hours. In small children a precordial and possibly an esophageal stethoscope is always recommendable.

Because of the special significance of pulse oxymetry and capnometry these will now be briefly discussed in more detail.

Pulse Oxymetry

This method combines the principles of spectrophotometric oxymetry and plethysmography. It uses a red light and an infrared light source and a receiver for electromagnetic radiation. Arterial pulsation and the degree of oxygenation produce characteristic fluctuations of light intensity. The registration of the arterial pulsation is the prerequisite for the recording.

This technique does not measure the fractional saturation, which is a measure of the oxygen load of all fractions of hemoglobin, but the functional saturation. This does not include CO-Hb and Met-Hb so that scientifically speaking, nonexact values are obtained. A heavy smoker has a fraction of 10 % CO-Hb after a couple

of inhalations of cigarette smoke. This would result in falsely high readings. The same applies for a CO intoxication. If the findings are confusing, an exact in-vitro measure of the arterial oxygen concentration should be resorted to. Calibration of the instrument is neither necessary nor possible and it is simple to use. The sensor is placed over a finger and 20–30 seconds after the instrument is switched on, a reading is obtained. The reliability of the measurements has been confirmed for all age groups, the only limitation being the absolute accuracy. The special value of pulse oxymetry for laser procedures lies in the assessment of patients during the use of an argon laser. The protective shields used for argon lasers make the clinical evaluation of the patient's skin color difficult, as they contain special integrated color filters.

Capnometry

Gases absorb electromagnetic radiation. The absorbed wavelengths are thereby specific for every gas. The infrared spectral analysis of CO_2 was first described in 1943. Light from an infrared light source is directed via mirror into a reference chamber with known gas content and via a second mirror into an analysis chamber with unknown CO_2 concentration. The light leaving the test chamber will be weaker than that leaving the reference chamber due to absorption by CO_2. The difference is proportional to the CO_2 concentration of the analyzed gas and this can be transformed into an electric signal (Braun and Fritz, 1994).

The measurement can be taken in the main gas stream and in the side stream. The latter is more commonly practiced in the clinical routine. Capnometry is a quantitatively exact measuring process and requires regular calibrations with a gas of known concentration. The interpretation of caponographical measurements in the clinical practice is not easy since they are influenced by ventilatory, circulatory, and metabolic factors. Metabolic changes occur slowly (hypothermia). Circulatory factors such as different forms of embolic disease or cardiac arrest result in an abrupt lowering or complete cessation of the reading. The normal value ranges between 5.0 % and 5.5 %. Variations of the measured value are usually due to ventilatory reasons in the form of hypercapnia or hypocapnia. A careful analysis is required for the individual case. Capnometry has become an indispensable component of patient monitoring during anesthesia. Anyone who has gained experience with this monitoring method will not want to miss it, as is the case with pulse oxymetry.

☞ Pulse oxymetry and capnometry should be used for patient monitoring.

Jet Ventilation

This technique has its beginnings in the development of the Sanders injector in 1967 and the method of high frequency jet ventilation (HFJV) by Sjöstrand in 1970 and Klain and Smith in 1977. Since these days this tube-free form of ventilation has carved a niche for itself in the surgical treatment of laryngeal and tracheal pathologies (Blomquist et al., 1990; Hirlinger et al., 1983; Hunton and Sowal, 1988; Jeckstrøm et al., 1992; Kurzeja et al., 1986; Mayne et al., 1991; Padfield and Stamp, 1992; Shikowitz et al., 1991). In the meantime a machine has become available that complies with the regulations for medical appliances and hence meets certain safety requirements, such as automatic switch-off of the gas supply when a rise in pressure occurs. This machine is the Acutronic MS 1000 (Stimotron, Wendelstein, Germany). It contains a microchip-controlled ventilator, a monitoring system for ventilating frequency, gas pressure, length of inspiratory cycle, tidal volume, and pressure limits and has an incorporated device for the humidification and warming of the inspired gas.

☞ The free gas flow from the bronchial tree is important for the clinical application. This must always be maintained.

Capnometry is not possible with this technique. In order to monitor the arterial partial pressure of CO_2 a blood gas analysis must be performed. Otherwise, a conventional respiratory cycle with capnometry must be interposed between two periods of jet ventilation. Intraoperative pulse oxymetry is necessary and the administration of muscle relaxants obligatory, although on principle the open system is conducive to spontaneous respiratory efforts. Clinical indications are in particular microsurgical laser procedures in the larynx and operations in the trachea. It can also be used for laryngoscopies and bronchoscopies. Jet ventilation is especially suited to shorter procedures, since regurgitation and aspiration cannot be excluded. The jet stream can be applied to the supraglottic or infraglottic airway (Fig. 4.**4**). The former is usually done through the laryngoscope. Care must be taken to direct the gas stream onto the glottic aperture as accurately as possible. Successful ventilation can be deducted from the oscillations of the thoracic wall in the rhythm of the chosen ventilating frequency. The rhythmic movements of the larynx are, however, unpleasant for the surgeon. Fortunately, these are less marked with infraglottic application of the jet stream, which is achieved by percutaneous cannulation of the trachea through the cricothyroid ligament (transtracheal jet ventilation) or infraglottic placement of the jet probe.

The Hunsaker Mon-Jet tube Fig. 4.**5** is a laser-safe, subglottic jet ventilation tube constructed of a non-

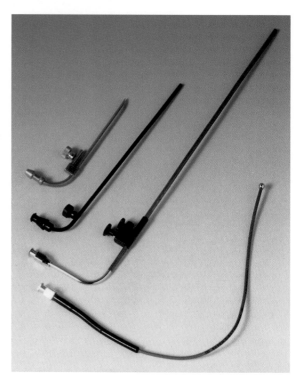

Fig. 4.**4**   Connecting pipes for transoral application of jet ventilation. To the left are three metal connectors which can be mounted directly onto the laryngoscope for the supraglottic application of the jet stream. The flexible pipe to the right is introduced infraglottically.

flammable fluoroplastic material. It allows monitoring of tracheal pressure and end tidal carbon dioxide, and it is designed with a basket-shaped distal extension to align the jet port away from the tracheal mucosa and to prevent trauma and submucosal injection of jetted gas.

The tip of the probe should be above the tracheal bifurcation. Humidification of the inspired gases must be considered for long-term use of the method in an intensive care setting. Intraoperatively it can, however, lead to an impairment of the surgeon's view.

Recommended settings for a young adult patient without underlying pulmonary disease are flow of 12–20 L/min, ventilating frequency of 100–150 per min, insufflation time of 30–40 % and a pressure of 0.7–2.1 bar. The gas exchange becomes insufficient for carbon dioxide when very high jet frequencies are reached. The

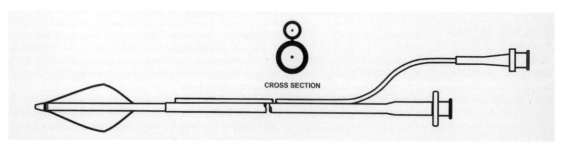

CROSS SECTION

Fig. 4.**5**   The Hunsaker Mon-Jet tube (Brooker et al, 24, 1998 [see text])

settings have to be individually adjusted for every case. Children and infants that are easily ventilated require much lower flows and pressure settings.

The complications are negligible if the technique of HFJV is used correctly and with care.

⚡ Lack of attention, especially to the passage for gas outflow, inappropriate anesthetic depth, lack of relaxation, and a displaced jet probe can lead to severe complications of barotrauma. These are pneumothorax, tension pneumothorax, mediastinal emphysema, inflation of the stomach, regurgitation, and aspiration. Long-term application of very dry gas can result in damage to the mucosa. An excessively high minute volume can lead to lowering of the mean arterial pressure due to a decrease of cardiac preload and an increased afterload. Contraindications for jet ventilation are markedly decreased compliance of lungs and thorax, severe bronchopulmonary and cardiovascular diseases, gross obesity, and a very advanced age.

Cuirass Ventilation

This constitutes an interesting alternative to other forms of ventilation. Cuirass ventilation functions according to the principle of negative pressures applied from the outside, similar to the concept of the iron lung. The thorax is completely surrounded by an armor, through which pressure changes can be applied (Fig. 4.**6**). The principle of cuirass ventilation is not new. What is new, however, is the possibility of using high frequencies for this, similar to jet ventilation (Dilkes et al., 1993). The advantage over jet ventilation is the security against barotrauma. Occasionally the insertion of a nasopharyngeal airway is necessary. First experiences with adult patients show that the technique can be used for laryngotracheal procedures that the optimal ventilating frequency is 120 per min and that vibrations in the operative field can occur similar to jet ventilation. We have not had any personal experience with this method, although the noninvasiveness makes this technique an interesting option.

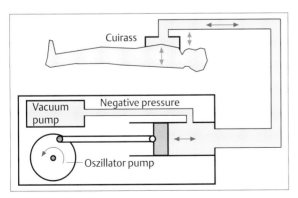

Fig. 4.**6** Schematic drawing of the cuirass ventilator. A piston pump creates pressure fluctuations which are transmitted to the lungs via an airtight thoracic armor.

Table 4.**3** Sequence of measures in case of fire or explosion. The actions listed under 2. and 3. should preferably be carried out simultaneously

1. Discontinuation of ventilation
2. Removal of all instrumentation and swabs
3. Extubation and fire extinction with saline
4. Ventilation via mask
5. Reintubation
6. Consolidation phase
7. Bronchoscopy

Ventilating Bronchoscopy

In certain, rare, situations the application of the CO_2 laser through the rigid ventilating bronchoscope becomes necessary. On principle this is only possible during shorter procedures. The ventilation is guaranteed by adequate depth of anesthesia, good relaxation, and a high gas flow. A cuff taken from a large-bore endotracheal tube can be sleeved over the bronchoscope and assist in the ventilation (Grant et al., 1993; Perera and Mallon, 1987). A flexible instrument for the application of Nd:YAG laser treatment can also be introduced via the rigid bronchoscope.

During the laser application an oxygen concentration of 40 % should not be exceeded and a short apneic phase used for the treatment. Rigid bronchoscopy can also be used in combination with HFJV.

Measures in Case of Fire

The careful adherence to the previously mentioned guidelines make incidences of fire or explosion very unlikely. If these complications occur, this is usually due to carelessness or lack of knowledge or experience. All personnel involved in laser surgery and in particular surgeons and anesthesiologists should be prepared for this situation. Certain successive measures must be familiar to all involved personnel and these must be carried out smoothly and swiftly (Table 4.**3**). The initial step must be to discontinue the ventilation in order to stop the oxygen flow to the site of the fire.

Any material or instrument inserted into the patient must be immediately removed. This includes the laryngoscope and the protective swabs and is due to the high temperatures that persist after the fire has been extinguished which are responsible for additional tissue damage. Ventilation is continued by mask. Subsequently the situation is stabilized and ventilation, oxygenation, circulation, and depth of anesthesia are controlled and optimized. Following this a bronchoscopy through a rigid endoscope is performed to assess the damage. If necessary, further foreign material and tissue particles are removed in the process. The decision on whether the operation can be continued or whether intensive therapeutic measures need to be initiated depends on the degree of thermal damage.

5 The Role of the Phoniatrician in Laser Surgery of the Larynx

Preoperative Period

Supplementary Functional Diagnosis

Endoscopic (video) laryngoscopy is performed to assess vocal cord mobility, tumor extent, and exact tumor localization. With appropriate experience in voice rehabilitation the compensatory level of phonation (glottic, ventricular, aryepiglottic) can already be estimated preoperatively. In some cases this postoperative substitute for previous phonation will already have developed spontaneously as a result of the disease process.

Endoscopic (video) stroboscopy can help in the assessment of the depth of infiltration of a tumor by analyzing the changes of the vibratory characteristics of the visible parts of the vocal folds or the parts of the cord that have not yet been infiltrated by tumor.

Good communication between phoniatrician and surgeon is of great importance and the surgeon must be informed about the findings of the phoniatric and stroboscopic assessment.

Preoperative Documentation

This consists of
– Videostroboscopy of the larynx,
– Endoscopic photography or laser printouts taken during quiet respiration and phonation.
In cases of benign lesions an objective voice assessment is made and a voice profile drawn up.

Preoperative Counseling of the Patient

The patient must be informed about the changes that are necessary for voice use and vocal hygiene during the postoperative period and the voice quality that is to be expected.

Absolute *voice rest* in the postoperative period is not mandatory for either benign or malignant lesions. For obvious reasons, this is also hardly achievable. Relative voice rest means that patients use their voice spontaneously as they did before the operation. If necessary, this must be demonstrated and practiced. However, patients must not whisper or strain their voice. The voice should only be used when absolutely necessary. Patients must be counseled and prepared to accept the resulting voice quality and alterations of vocal characteristics (hoarseness, aphonia).

After surgery for malignant tumors, a tissue defect usually occurs in the operated area which prevents contact during phonation. Voice protection should not be exaggerated in these cases. On the contrary, the spontaneous attempts to phonate often result in the development of a quite useful *compensatory mechanism,* which can be used for further voice rehabilitation. Wound healing is improved by saline inhalations. Chamomile should be avoided and other added medications are not necessary. It is important to discuss with the patient the fact that, independent of the preservation of the larynx, the voice is also spared in the procedure.

Postoperative Check-ups

Control Before Discharge

The postoperative phonation is assessed laryngoscopically and, if necessary, stroboscopically. Concrete instructions are given with regard to correct voice habits. If healing problems are encountered during recovery of the patient, further controls may be indicated.

Control After Completion of Wound Healing

Diagnosis of Function

Endoscopic (video) laryngoscopy is used to assess the remaining defect, the contact on phonation, compensatory mechanisms of phonation, scar formation, and possible synechiae.

Endoscopic (video) stroboscopy analyses the quality of the vibrations, phonatory closure phase, and contact. It is not performed in aphonic patients.

Objective voice assessment of sustained phonation as well as running speech (e.g., "rainbow passage") is part of the check-up (Fröhlich et al., in press). Vocal parameters that are routinely assessed are pitch, loudness, quality, breath features, and rate. The fundamental frequency is analyzed, as are pitch pertubation (jitter) and amplitude pertubation (shimmer). Further, the noise-to-harmonic ratio (NHR), the voice turbulence index (VTI), and the glottal-to-noise-excitation ratio (GNE) (Michaelis et al, 1997) can be used in the assessment. Other methods of analysis include dynamic range analysis and aerodynamic tests (mean flow rate and glottal airflow).

Perceptual or subjective voice analysis is also part of the routine assessment of all patients and supplements the objective voice analysis.

Postoperative Documentation

– Endoscopic laryngoscopy and stroboscopy with video and audio documentation;
– Endoscopic photography or laser prints of glottis in respiration and phonation;
– Objective voice analysis;
– Perceptual voice analysis including recordings.

Advice on Voice Use and Vocal Straining

After wound healing has been completed, voice protection is no longer justifiable. An exception is an intercurrent acute laryngitis. The different ways of voice straining must be explained and distinguished from voice abuse. The phenomenon of perilaryngeal paresthesias must be discussed with the patient. These comprise globus sensation, dry feeling in the throat, local pain, or pain radiating to the ear or mastoid, and may lead to habitual throat clearing. The symptoms usually vary with the use of the voice. Advice should be given on the symptomatic treatment with regular saline inhalations for a maximum of 2–3 weeks.

Advice on Voice Rehabilitation

Video recordings of the individual patient can help to illustrate the problem and explain the desired results. The *aim* is an optimal compensatory phonation technique for the individual patient.

The *chances* of achieving this depend greatly on the physical condition of the patient, age, motivation, and compliance with the treatment.

The employed *method* is that of functional voice therapy (Kruse, 1989; Kruse, 1991; Kruse 1998), based on the concept of the laryngeal double valve function (Jacoby, 1987; Rabine, 1987; Rohmert, 1987).

The *intensity* of the rehabilitation depends on the individual. On average, two individual sessions per weekday are held over a period of 2–4 weeks.

The *organization* of the therapy depends on the distance between the patient's home and the therapy center. Daily visits from home may be considered, or alternatively intensive treatment during a stay in a hotel or even admission for rehabilitation need to be planned. Fees and payment have to be discussed and arranged beforehand.

Stage of Voice Rehabilitation

- Initial diagnostic procedures and documentation (identical to p. 124);
- Reassessments and documentation in the postoperative period every 14 days, depending on the individual and encountered difficulties;
- Final assessment and documentation (identical to p. 124).

In the final session between patient, phoniatrician, and speech pathologist the achieved results of voice quality and the individual limits of vocal straining are discussed. Instructions for vocal hygiene and home exercises are given and the date for the next check-up is fixed, usually in 2–3 months. Effects of additional diseases of the larynx on the voice should also be mentioned (acute laryngitis, voice abuse). If necessary, the special requirements for reentry into the job market and other particular phonatory challenges are discussed.

Results of Vocal Function

A certain relationship between the extent of the minimally invasive resection and the level of phonation which can be achieved by voice rehabilitation is becoming evident. Knowledge of the physiology and pathophysiology (Kruse, 1989; Kruse, 1991; Kruse, 1998) of voice production based on the concept of the double valve function of the larynx (Jacoby, 1987; Kruse, 1989; Kruse, 1991; Kruse, 1998; Rabine, 1987; Rohmert, 1987) is thereby helpful. Naturally, any form of posttherapeutic phonation can only be a *compensatory form of voice production* and not a normal voice. This is caused by the destruction of normal morphology, which is inevitable in the process of curative resections.

The best functional results are obtained from a compensatory phonation produced at the level of the *vocal folds* (Fig. 5.**7**). In our experience this can be achieved after unilateral or bilateral partial cordectomy. If the depth of the resection is not more than 5 mm, even the vibratory characteristics of the operated vocal fold are regained. The second best result of vocal function is achieved by *ventricular* phonation (Kruse, 1981) as substitute for the normal voice. This voice is aimed for following total cordectomy and additional partial resection of one or both ventricular folds, should this have been necessary for oncological reasons. If this level can also not be utilized due to the extent of the resection, vocal compensation at an *aryepiglottic* level finally remains. This compensatory aryepiglottic voice is adequate for purposes of social communication and may even be sufficient for the workplace under specific acoustic conditions and for certain degrees of strain that are required from the voice. One of our patients even had his pilot's licence reissued, which included a radio licence. He had a recurrent T3 tumor after previous radiotherapy elsewhere which was then resected by laser.

Supraglottic vocal compensatory mechanisms usually develop spontaneously with postoperative voice use. In these cases rehabilitation is mostly necessary to *optimize* the dynamic and technical aspects. Whether a ventricular voice can be changed back to the glottic level depends on surgical factors, as assessed by the phoniatrician, and the rehabilitative method and approach. To our knowledge this specific manipulation of the different levels of phonation is only possible in a regular fashion by the use of our concept of *"functional voice therapy"* (Kruse, 1989; Kruse, 1991; Kruse, 1998). No qualitatively and quantitatively comparable results are available from other conservative surgical strategies or reconstructive procedures.

Postrehabilitation Period

- Diagnostic procedures for control purposes and documentation (identical to p. 124);
- Individual advice on voice use.

If necessary, the decision to repeat the rehabilitation program must be made.

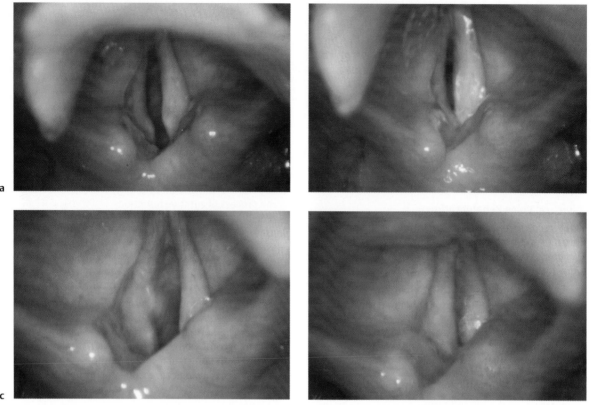

Fig. 5.**1** Glottic compensatory phonation (vocal folds). After partial left-sided cordectomy (pT1 with maximum depth of infiltration of 3 mm) before (**a** and **b**) and after voice reha-bilitation (**c** and **d**). Laryngoscopically the improved closure and almost normal contour of the vocal fold can be recognized. Compensation by the ventricular folds has been reduced.

Operative Prerequisites for Phoniatric Aftercare

Certain surgical factors are prerequisites for the achievement of the optimal results of vocal function for the individual patient. These are mainly:

– Minimally invasive resection if it is oncologically justifiable;
– Surgical planning although primarily concerned about oncological principles should take the laryngeal levels of phonation (glottic, ventricular, aryepiglottic) into account;
– Preservation of laryngeal innervation. This will prevent muscular atrophy and maximum use can be made of residual mobility;
– A two- or better three-dimensional graphic report on the performed resection. This helps in the planning of the postoperative rehabilitation program.

Final Comments

As has been shown, a close cooperation must be maintained between otorhinolaryngologist and phoniatrician in planning, performing, and aftercare of minimally invasive laryngeal surgery. This helps to not only reduce the extent of the functional voice problems that become manifest in the immediate postoperative phase, but also favorably influences the further course by applying the measures of voice rehabilitation.

By comparison, an unusually high quality of life ensues, as swallowing and respiratory functions of the larynx are almost always unaffected. Furthermore, an improved and sometimes almost normal vocal function allows for a smooth reintegration into the patient's social and, if pertinent, occupational life. For these reasons the voice rehabilitation techniques should be used as vigorously as for any dysphonia of another cause.

Quantitative and qualitative standards are set for postoperative voice quality and function by the cases documented herein. They can serve as a basis for comparative multi-center studies and for evaluation of alternative concepts. Apart from the obligatory oncological results and statistics of tumor survival, any future treatment concept will have to satisfy the requirements and *norms of postoperative functional quality*. Our preoperative estimation of possible postoperative voice quality makes it possible for us to counsel the realistic expectations of the patient regarding voice function.

Examples of Results

1. Endoscopic photos of different levels of compensatory phonation (Fig. 5.**1**–5.**5**).
2. Results of acoustic voice analyses (Fig. 5.**6**–5.**8**).

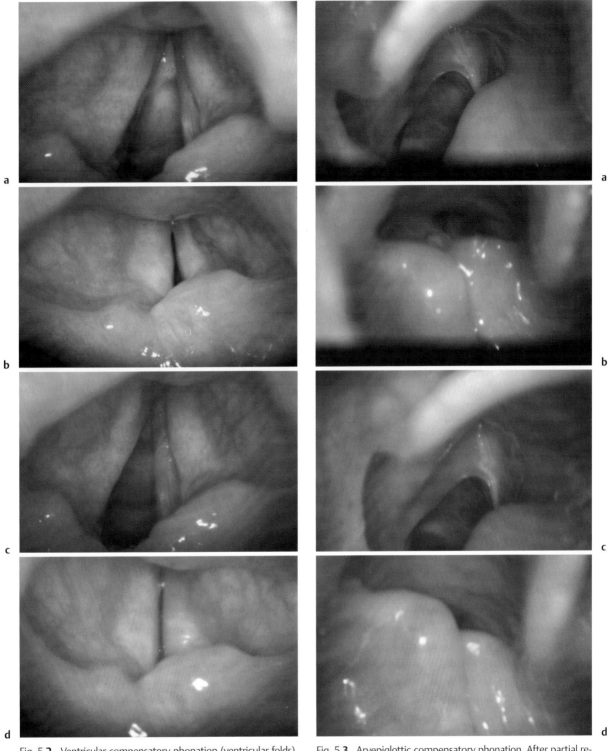

Fig. 5.**2** Ventricular compensatory phonation (ventricular folds). After nearly total left-sided cordectomy (T1 with a maximum depth of infiltration of 5 mm) before (**a** and **b**) and after voice rehabilitation (**c** and **d**). Apart from the improved closure of the ventricular folds, the effects of voice rehabilitation can be seen in the larger anteroposterior aperture of the supraglottis. This is the result of less straining during phonation and improved sound transmission.

Fig. 5.**3** Aryepiglottic compensatory phonation. After partial resection of a pT3 tumor on the right side. The maximum depth of infiltration was 10 mm and 7 mm in the areas of the vocal fold and the ventricular fold respectively. The anterior part of the left vocal fold also had to be resected. Before (**a** and **b**) and after (**c** and **d**) voice rehabilitation. Postoperatively an interarytenoid level of phonation formed spontaneously. This was changed by voice rehabilitation to a phonatory contact between left aryepiglottic fold and laryngeal surface of the epiglottis (petiole). (See Fig. 3.**29**. This is the same patient after wound healing has been completed.)

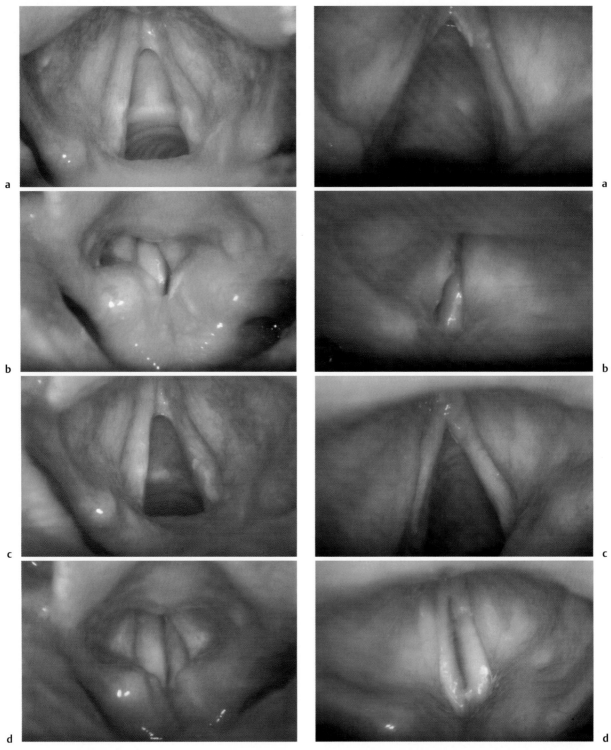

Fig. 5.**4** Glottoventricular compensatory phonation (phonatio obliqua; Kleinsasser et al., 1975). This special form of compensation mechanism is mostly only found immediately postoperatively (**a** and **b**). Here the approximation of right ventricular fold and left vocal fold is visible. In this case a partial resection of the right vocal fold with inclusion of the anterior commissure was performed (pT1 with maximum depth of infiltration of 3 mm). Synechia formation was slight. After rehabilitation (**c** and **d**) a glottic compensatory mechanism became manifest.

Fig. 5.**5** Shift of voice production level through rehabilitative measures. This patient had a bilateral partial cordectomy with resection of the anterior commissure (pT1b with maximum depth of infiltration of 2 mm). Postoperatively a ventricular compensation mechanism developed spontaneously (**a** and **b**). This was changed to a functionally superior glottic level of phonation (**c** and **d**). The small keratotic lesion on the free margin of the right vocal fold has subsequently been removed. The patient has been free of disease for 7 years.

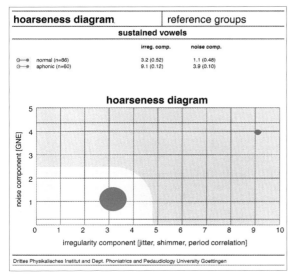

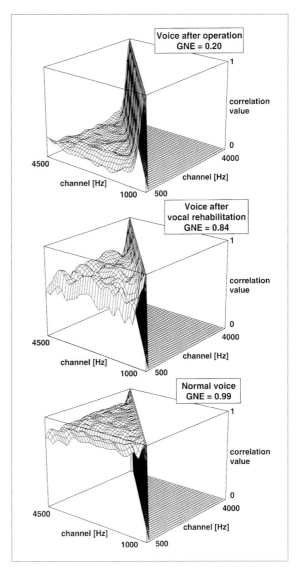

Voice after operation
GNE = 0.20

correlation
value

channel [Hz]

channel [Hz]

Voice after
vocal rehabilitation
GNE = 0.84

correlation
value

channel [Hz]

channel [Hz]

Normal voice
GNE = 0.99

correlation
value

channel [Hz]

channel [Hz]

Fig. 5.6 Voice analysis by the Göttingen Hoarseness Diagram. The parameters for voice quality analysis are irregularity component plotted on the x-axis and noise component on the y-axis. The extremes of "normal voice" (green) and "aphonia" (red) are shown.

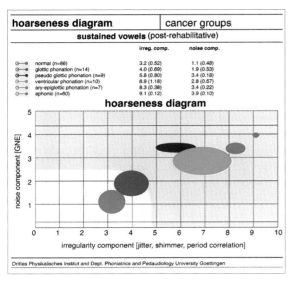

Fig. 5.8 Quantitative improvement of the GNE factor (Pressman, 1954; Rabine, 1987) from 0.31 postoperatively to 0.89 after voice rehabilitation (normal value 0.998). This was achieved by changing the level from a ventricular phonation technique that had formed spontaneously after the operation to a glottic voice (see Fig. 5.5). Compared to any other analysis system, this parameter of voice quality developed by our group can even be measured in cases of severe hoarseness or aphonia.

Fig. 5.7 This shows current results of our efforts with functional voice rehabilitation. An obvious system of voice quality grading becomes evident after minimally invasive laser resections of glottic carcinomas. Vocal compensation on a glottic level results in less hoarseness than ventricular or aryepiglottic mechanisms. Ventricular compensation techniques sometimes demonstrate less noise component than a pseudoglottic technique in which no vibration of the operated vocal fold was achieved through rehabilitative measures. As expected the aryepiglottic vocal compensation shows the greatest degree of hoarseness.

6 Laser Physics and Laser Safety

Introduction to Laser Physics

Lasers are a relatively new component of surgical equipment. There is still significant ignorance by the medical profession in general about laser physics and the interaction of lasers and tissues. A basic knowledge of laser physics is thus not only required for the safe operation of laser equipment in the operating room, but also to enable the surgeon to counsel the patient appropriately.

Electromagnetic radiation has become indispensable in modern medicine and is assuming a pivotal role particularly in diagnosis and therapy. Daily reminders of this are radiographs, which are used in imaging, including computed tomography (CT), ionizing radiation used in radiotherapy, high frequency and IR radiation in thermotherapy, phototherapy with or without biologically active photosensitisers and, last but not least, the cold-light illumination of the operative field in and outside the body.

Electromagnetic radiation can be divided into ionizing and nonionizing radiation. Although other forms of radiation are used in radiography and radiotherapy, the most important source of electromagnetic energy in medicine is ionizing radiation with a very short wave length, i.e., X-rays and gamma radiation. Light from the ultraviolet (UV) to the IR part of the spectrum does not generally have an ionizing effect. This is also true of the lasers used in surgery.

Surgical lasers work by transforming radiation energy into heat at the incident spot. In this respect the laser can be compared to an electrocautery probe. The difference is that the laser is generally not applied by direct contact between the tissue and the probe. Instead, it strikes the tissue in the form of focused radiation. The point of interaction between laser and tissue results in intense local heat production.

The light of the laser has the same physical characteristics as "normal" visible light. It can be reflected by mirrors and it can be focused through lenses. In comparison to light from conventional sources, however, the laser beam is collimated (coherent), it is of a single wavelength (monochromatic) and is powerful.

The light of UV or IR lasers is invisible to the human eye. Hence, the point where the beam of medically used UV or IR lasers hits the tissue's surface must be marked. For this purpose a visible aiming laser beam is used coaxially with the invisible working laser.

Properties of Laser Light

The most important properties that characterize a laser beam are: the laser wavelength, the beam divergence, the size of the focal spot, the beam profile, the power density, and the energy density within the spot.

Wavelength

The wavelength corresponds to the color of the light. It is measured in nanometer (nm) or micrometer (µm): 1 µm is equal to 1000 nm. Visible light has a spectrum between 400 nm (violet) and 750 nm (red). Excimer lasers emit UV radiation of between 193 nm and 351 nm. Visible laser light is, for instance, produced by Argon lasers (blue-green), dye lasers (adjustable within certain ranges of color), Alexandrite lasers (red), frequency doubled Nd:YAG lasers, sometimes called KTP lasers (green), Krypton lasers (red) and He-Ne lasers (red). Infrared lasers include Nd:YAG lasers (1064 nm), Holmium:YAG lasers (2100 nm), Erbium:YAG lasers (2900 nm) and CO_2 lasers (10 600 nm).

Divergence

Divergence is the angle at which the emitted laser beam opens up after leaving the laser device (Fig. 6.**1**). It is expressed as the ratio of the beam diameter to the distance from the laser source and is measured in radian (rad) or milliradian (mrad; 1/1000 rad). 1 mrad translates into a diameter of the beam of 10 mm at a distance of 10 m from the laser aperture.

The focus diameter is proportional to the angle of divergence of the laser beam and to the focal length of the lens used to focus the beam. The divergence is smallest when the laser operates in the fundamental mode. Fundamental mode lasers therefore provide the smallest focal spot sizes possible. According to physical laws, the angle of divergence increases with increasing laser wavelength. The CO_2 laser is the laser with the largest wavelength of all medically used lasers, namely 10,6 µm. This is the reason why it is not possible for the beam of a CO_2 laser to have a very small focal spot and at the same time to provide a great depth of focus. However, the best results are obtained with CO_2 lasers which operate in the fundamental mode (TEM 00).

Focal Spot Size

The almost parallel laser beam can be focused with a lens onto a small area which is called focal spot (Fig. 6.**2**). As in photography, there is a focal depth. This

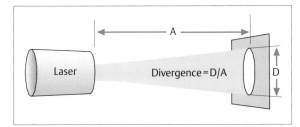

Fig. 6.**1** Divergence is the ratio of diameter D to length A of a laser beam.

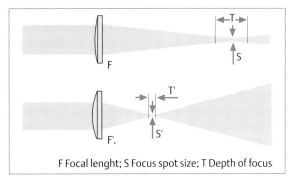

F Focal lenght; S Focus spot size; T Depth of focus

Fig. 6.**2** Focusing of the laser beam for two different focal lengths F and F'.

is the distance throughout which the beam remains focused after converging and before diverging. This depth is called the waist of the beam. The smaller the size of the focal spot produced by the lens, the shorter the focal depth. This means in practice that the tissue has to be more accurately positioned when a small focal spot is produced using a short focal length lens. The focal depth is a function of the square of the focal spot size. When a lens with half the focal length is chosen, this immediately translates into a focal spot of half the size. The focal depth then decreases to only one quarter. The respective data for the CO_2 laser are given in Table 6.**1**.

Beam Profile and Modes

These terms refer to the distribution of radiant energy across the beam diameter. The following different modes with their typical distribution of beam intensity are distinguished (see Fig. 6.**3**).

Fundamental mode. Alternative terms are TEM 00, Gaussian beam, and single mode. In this mode the highest power density is found at the centre of the beam. It decreases toward the periphery similar to a bell-shaped curve. It is the laser beam in this fundamental mode which can be focused onto the smallest possible spot. It is technically very demanding to obtain high power output from a laser operating in the fundamental mode. Most medical CO_2 lasers available today provide fundamental mode characteristics.

Multimode. Multimode lasers provide higher energy levels than lasers operating in the fundamental mode. They can, however, not be focused so sharply. Solid-state lasers, for instance, function in multimode to achieve an optimal power output. Laser radiation which is transmitted via flexible fibre optics also has multimode characteristics. The argon laser, for example, can

be used via a split lamp opthalmic microscope. Due to its short wavelength, however, it can still produce a sufficiently small spot on the retina of approximately 50 µm.

Ringmode (TEM 01). This is a special form of a mode which resembles the shape of a donut cake.

Waveguide mode. This mode is comparable to the fundamental mode. It is produced by so-called waveguide lasers. There are certain CO_2 lasers which work in the waveguide mode.

Power and Energy

These two factors are important for assessing the properties of the laser beam together with the output characteristics, namely continuous wave (CW) or pulsed use. The mathematical relation between power and energy is as follows: energy = power · exposure time.

Energy is measured in joules (J), power is measured in watts (W), and the exposure time is given in seconds (s). The power of *CW lasers* is determined by the power output of the laser. If the exposure time is set to a quarter of a second, for instance, then the applied energy can be calculated, as described, by multiplying power times exposure time.

Table 6.**1** The depth of focus, defined as the area where the beam diameter is less than 1.1 times the size of the spot at the waist of the beam. It increases proportionally to the square of the spot size

Spot size (mm)	0.1	0.2	0.5	1	2
Depth of focus (mm)	0.68	2.72	17	68	272

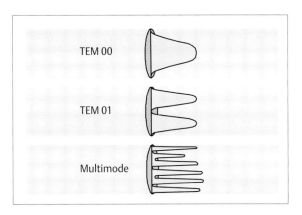

Fig. 6.**3** Mode profiles.

Pulsed lasers emit their energy by sending discrete impulses. The peak power can be calculated if the impulse duration is known by dividing the impulse energy by the impulse duration. Maximum power output can be very high, i.e., billions of watts, if the impulse is very short, i.e., a billionth of a second. The CO_2 lasers which are commonly used in surgery are normally operated in CW. Some lasers provide a so-called superpulse mode of operation. Superpulse lasers emit several thousand bursts of power per second. The peak power of the bursts which are achieved with the superpulse is a few hundred watts, although the average power is much smaller — it is the average power which the surgeon sets at the panel.

Irradiance and Radiant Exposure

The effects that a laser beam of certain power (or energy) has on the tissue depends on the area over which this power (or energy) is distributed. The biological effects are basically the same for the same irradiance. Irradiance is measured in W/m^2; radiant exposure is given in J/m^2.

The irradiances employed in surgery vary from ten to a few hundred million W/m^2.

Physics of the CO_2 Laser

The CO_2 laser beam is produced in a gas-containing discharge tube. The laser gas consists of a mixture of CO_2, He, and N, there are open and sealed-off laser designs. The sealed-off tube houses the gas mixture forever which is necessary for the operation of the laser. The open laser design implements a constant flow of laser gas coming from an external gas container. There is no need to exchange pressurized laser gas containers when the laser is a sealed type.

Sealed-off laser tubes set high demands for the tightness of the seals and the cleanness of the components during their assembly. Development today is so advanced that practically only sealed laser tube designs are offered with CO_2 lasers.

Some laser tubes are powered by electrical discharge of direct current; in others the energy is provided by the application of radio frequency fields.

The Beam Guiding System of the CO_2 Laser

The optics guiding the laser beam usually consists of a beam transmitter and a beam applicator.

The laser beam can be manipulated through the transmission unit. In the case of the CO_2 laser, mirrors on articulated arms are used for this purpose.

Beam applicators comprise handpieces, micro-manipulators, waveguide probes, and adapters for endoscopes.

Articulated Mirror Arm

The articulated mirror arm consists of straight tubes, angled pieces of tubing, and rotating bearings (Fig. 6.5). The angle pieces contain mirrors which are placed at an angle of 45°. Most arms have seven mirrors and seven articulating angle pieces. This arm design guarantees a full range of movement of the laser beam in all possible directions. There are other laser systems in which the laser head itself is movable. In these cases five articulations are adequate to achieve the full range of movements.

The precision of the articulations, their tolerance, and the precision of the mirror adjustments must be of the highest standards. The user must therefore take great care when maneuvering the arms. If the mirror arm is only bent by a few millimeters, disturbances in the form of shadows and scattering of the laser beam can occur.

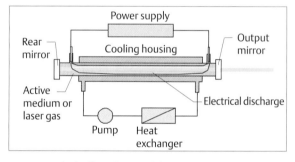

Fig. 6.4 Sealed-off CO_2 laser with basic components.

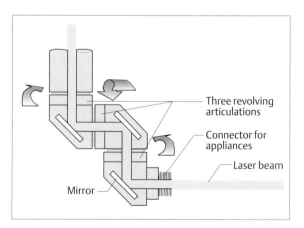

Fig. 6.5 Schematics of the articulations of a mirror arm for a CO_2 laser.

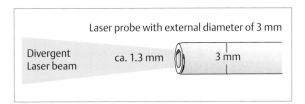

Fig. 6.**6** Tip of a waveguide probe. The laser beam diverges as it leaves the probe.

Beam Applicators

The surgeon directs the laser beam onto the tissue with the help of the beam applicator. The simplest applicator is the focusing handpiece. Apart from this, there are couplers for a number of optic instruments. These include adapters for operating microscopes, laparoscopes, bronchoscopes, etc.

There are also thin transmission probes for the radiation of the CO_2 laser. Ceramic capillaries which are continuously flushed with gas transmit the CO_2 laser beam by repeatedly reflecting it on their inner surface. The radiation of the laser is finally released from the end of the capillary at an angle of divergence of approximately 10°. The capillaries are kept clean by continuously flushing them with gas. Such transmission probes are rather rigid. They can be used in body cavities provided that they are inflated with gas and that straight access to the cavity is possible.

Micromanipulators are used during laser microsurgery. The laser focus can be moved around in the visual field manipulating a small control lever which is attached to the micromanipulator. Another control element allows the adjustment of the focus along the axis of the beam to the various focal lengths of the microscope. The optical system of a micromanipulator is shown in Fig. 6.**7**.

Modern micromanipulator controls have spot sizes of 0.2 mm diameter. They make it necessary to accurately position the operating microscope to within millimeters of the operated tissue, otherwise the beam is defocused, causing the cutting effect of the laser almost to be lost. Power settings of only a few watts are

adequate for dissections using this small spot size. Additionally, the collateral thermal damage to tissue is absolutely minimal.

A good compromise of the cutting ability, the spot size, and a comfortable depth of focus should be provided by micromanipulators producing a spot size of 0.5–0.8 mm.

Laser Tissue Interactions

When lasers were introduced into surgery in the years 1975–1980, they were primarily used as a new form of scalpel. A laser handpiece was used for plastic procedures. Subsequently, it became evident that the greatest benefit of the laser lies in minimally invasive surgery. Surgeons gained access to the operative site through loupes, stereoscopic microscopes, and through rigid or flexible endoscopes.

The laser ideally complements endoscopic instruments due to its unique advantages: high precision, easy manipulation, optimal effects on the tissue, and a no-touch surgical technique. There are lasers which work by producing photobiological, photodisruptive, or thermal effects. The CO_2 laser belongs to the category in which all energy is transformed into thermal energy. This heat is produced by the absorption of laser energy by the tissue.

Absorption

The tissue characteristic of greatest importance to laser medicine is the absorption of radiation. This effect depends on the wavelength of the laser. The tissues of the human body contain at least three components which differ significantly in their absorption characteristics. These are water, hemoglobin, and pigment (melanin). Fig. 6.**8** shows the depths of penetration of electromagnetic radiation in water and in a solution of hemoglobin.

The example of green light with a wavelength of approximately 0.5 µm demonstrates that this light is well absorbed by blood (hemoglobin) and penetrates only a short distance into the solution. Water, on the other hand, hardly absorbs green light at all. Green light obviously has a selective effect on blood. In surgical practice this means that the green light of the argon laser can be used by the surgeon to selectively heat up blood vessels and thus coagulate and seal them.

The knowledge of the penetrating powers of laser radiation are of immense importance for surgeons. The degree of penetration is directly dependent on the absorption properties of the target. Tissue layers which avidly absorb radiation prevent its further passage and therefore shield deeper lying regions.

It follows that the greater the absorption, the smaller the depth of penetration.

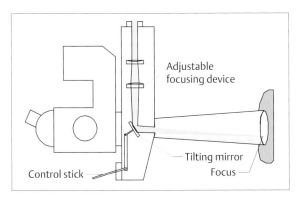

Fig. 6.**7** Micromanipulator.

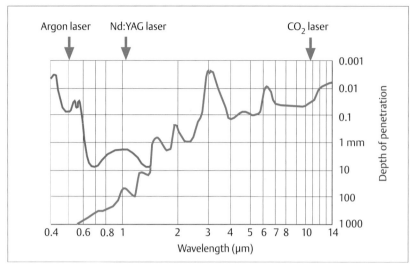

Fig. 6.8 Depth of penetration of electromagnetic radiation as function of its wavelength. A logarithmic scale is used for x- and y-axis. The red curve shows the depth of penetration into a solution of hemoglobin; light of short wavelength (green) as emitted by an argon laser hardly penetrates the solution and is therefore also effectively absorbed by blood within the vessels. The blue graph shows that the radiation of the CO_2 laser with a long wavelength of around 10 µm is quickly absorbed by water, the main component of tissues. This explains the limited depth of penetration of the CO_2 laser into tissue. (The red curve is only depicted for wavelengths up to 1.5 µm; the slope for greater wavelengths is practically identical to that of water.)

Radiation Scatter

Biological tissues scatter radiation with the exception of the transparent structures of the eye. The intensity of the radiation decreases with increasing tissue depth due to this scattering. A fraction of the radiation reaches beyond the spot's periphery, possibly causing some biological effect even there.

The phenomenon of scattering is greatly dependent on the wavelength. Radiation with a short wavelength is subjected to much greater scatter than radiation of longer wavelengths. Strong absorption limits the effect of scattering, since absorbed radiation can no longer be scattered.

Radiation scattering is therefore only of significance if the radiation has a short wavelength and is poorly absorbed.

In situations where there is more marked scattering, the laser radiation is also diffusely reflected to some extent. Remittance is the proportion of the incident radiation which is lost due to diffuse reflection by the various layers of tissue. In the case of the Nd:YAG laser remittance can be up to one third of the incident level of radiation.

The effects of scattering and of reflectance are of no practical importance when CO_2 lasers are used.

Thermal Conduction

The actual purpose of laser energy in medicine is to locally produce heat on the tissue surfaces. The thermal energy is then used surgically to cut, vaporize, or coagulate tissue.

Any material has the tendency to conduct heat toward the periphery if there are areas within it that have a higher temperature than the surroundings. Thermal energy is then transmitted from the warm to the cold areas. This process continues until the temperature is the same everywhere. The smaller the heated area, the more quickly the exchange of temperature takes place. In practice this means a quicker cooling-off period for laser radiation where the laser wavelength provides only shallow penetration and where a small focal spot is chosen.

The surrounding of the laser spot is heated by thermal conduction. Prolonged time of exposure of a heavily absorbed laser radiation like that of the CO_2 laser can result in thermally affecting the close vicinity of the laser spot. This thermal zone is typically only a fraction of a millimeter wide if the laser time was a few seconds long. It can become a few millimeters wide if the laser was defocused and the radiation lasted for some minutes.

This concludes the discussion of the most basic physical principles which are important for laser medicine. Lasers are particularly suited for the manipulation of the parameters of the radiation in order to achieve the desired thermal effects on the tissues. The range of possible applications of lasers on tissue stretches from the thermal denaturation of disease processes of a few millimetres in size to precise surgical procedures on extended structures, including the most delicate microsurgical preparations, for example, on small blood vessels and nerves.

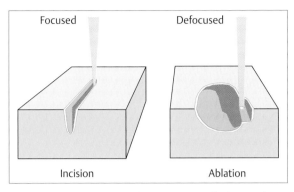

Fig. 6.**9** Tissue ablation and transection with the CO_2 laser.

Thermal Effects on Tissue

Depending on the amount of thermal energy applied to the tissue, the following effects can be observed:
– 45°C: reversible interference with cellular metabolism (edema zone).
– 50°C: irreversible thermal cell damage.
– 60°C: protein denatures; the tissue coagulates, blood darkens.
– 80°C: collagen fibers contract; tissue shrinks; vessels shrink.
– 100°C: the water content of tissue evaporates; craters form, edges desiccate.
– 250°C: tissue disintegrates and carbonizes.

The different therapeutic aims are:
– Thermal denaturation of tumor tissue (60°C),
– Coagulation of blood vessels (80–100°C),
– Ablation of tissue by vaporization (100°C and above).

In certain cases the thermal damage must be minimized as in microsurgery. In other situations deep thermal penetration is desired, for example, for the thermal denaturation of extensive tumors. In the first case laser radiation is chosen which is easily absorbed and which is additionally applied in pulsed mode in order to minimize thermal conduction. The CO_2 laser, preferably set to the superpulse mode, is well suited for this purpose. In the second case a Nd:YAG laser may be a better choice.

The CO_2 laser is the laser system with the greatest impact on otorhinolaryngological practice. The effects and applications of the CO_2 laser are discussed in the following section.

Effects and Applications of the CO_2-Laser

Effects

The wavelength of the CO_2 laser is 10.6 μm. It lies in the far IR spectrum. This wavelength is absorbed by almost all materials. Exceptions are metals which reflect IR radiation or other special materials which transmit the radiation of this wavelength. The laser radiation is readily absorbed by the most superficial layer of biological materials; penetration is negligible. There is almost no scattering. The power of the incident laser beam is transformed into heat within a very small tissue volume. Thus, the power per unit of volume is very high. During the short impulses of the superpulsed emission which last for only a few milliseconds, the boiling point of water is reached. The incident radiation evaporates the tissue water and leads to a sudden release of nonliquid particles which take the form of a laser plume.

If the laser is applied continuously to a certain target area, a crater forms of increasing depth. The edges of the crater are thereby heated up to 100°C and the adjacent tissue is affected by thermal conduction. However, with the commonly used technique of laser application there is hardly any spread of thermal energy toward the structures surrounding the target tissue.

In the region around the zone of vaporization or ablation, small blood vessels are closed off. The resulting desiccated surface layer seems to effectively seal the adjacent tissue. This mechanism seems to successfully prevent the invasion of infectious agents and the loss of tissue fluids.

Applications

The operative techniques employing the CO_2 laser make use of these special properties in the following way:
- Tissue ablation with beam diameters between 1–4 mm. The incident laser radiation is kept on the tissue that needs to be resected until it has been completely vaporized.
- Tissue transection (incision). The diameters of the focus are chosen between 0.2–1 mm. The laser beam is used like a scalpel.

The surgical procedures which allow the CO_2 laser to be used to its full advantage are the bloodless or almost bloodless removal of tissue. This is mainly achieved by the simultaneous coagulation of small blood vessels. The laser beam can be manipulated under microscopic or endoscopic control with greatest precision, while the view of the area of dissection remains unimpaired.

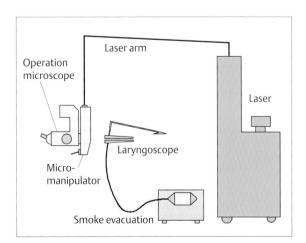

Fig. 6.**10** Microsurgical workplace.

Instruments and Laser Workplace

CO$_2$ Laser

– Power: at least 30 W, 40–60 W are recommended;
– Superpulse to minimize thermal damage and the effect of carbonization;
– Operation in a closed system;
– Adequate range and overhead assembly of the laser arm;
– Simple operation;
– The microscope with connected laser should be able to swing away from the operative field.

Micromanipulator Control

Optical:
– Focusing on a distance of 400 mm;
– Defocusing possible to a diameter of approximately 3 mm;
– Good axial alignment of the aiming beam and working laser beam;
– Focus size 0.5–0.8 mm.

Mechanical:
– Effortless, precise control of the focal spot;
– No lagging of the focal spot behind the manipulating lever movements, i.e., no hysteresis;
– Least possible obstruction of view;
– No parallax, i.e., the axis of the laser beam should be coincident with the microscope's axis of view.

Smoke Evacuation

The smoke evacuation system serves to remove the smoke and plumes which present potential health hazards. It also helps to keep a clear field of vision. The scavenging system for anesthetic gases which is installed in the operating room is suitable for the evacuation of the tissue plume if a filter is installed to keep out larger particles. Surgical suction systems do not have incorporated smoke filters.

Special smoke evacuators are available on the market. They should fulfill the *demands* of
– Sufficient vacuum to effectively suck the smoke through the narrow pipes integrated in the laryngoscope,
– Low noise levels.

Laser Safety

The safety aspect of lasers and their use is stipulated in governmental regulations. The system safety refers to design and manufacture of the laser product and its use. In the United States its features are mandated under the Radiation Control for Health and Safety Act of 1968. The product must meet these requirements and must be certified with the Center for Devices and Radiological Health (CDRH) of the Food and Drug Administration (FDA).

Guidelines on safe practices and occupational exposure limits are laid down by the Laser Institute of America along with the Committee Z136 of the American National Standards Institute in the American National Standard for the Safe Use of Lasers in Health Care Facilities (ANSI Z136.3 of 1996).

In other countries, national regulations about laser safety are in effect and should be followed by the laser user.

The International Electrotechnical Commission (IEC) has prepared the "Guide for the Safe Use of Medical Laser Equipment," IEC 60825-8, published in 1999, (IEC, 3 rue de Varembé, Genève, Switzerland).

Laser radiation is hazardous for several reasons:
• Laser beams of the visible or near IR part of the spectrum are focused by the refractive media of the eye. Very small powers as low as some milliwatts are sufficient to cause damage to the retina. Lasers with wavelengths in the middle and far IR spectrum damage the cornea.

Table 6.**2** Checklist of safety measures for laser use in the operating room

Item	Safety measures
1.	Appoint a laser safety officer
2.	Provide laser safety training to health care personnel
3.	Set up and follow standard operating procedures
4.	Label entrances to laser treatment rooms
5.	Install warning lights at the entrances to laser treatment rooms
6.	Make laser protective eye wear available
7.	Apply prophylactic measures against fire
8.	Apply prophylactic measures against toxic fumes
9.	Provide laser, safety eyewear
10.	Train the staff annually
11.	Prevent fire
12.	Remove hazardous laser plume

- Some laser radiation is invisible to the human eye. The aversion response of the eye, which otherwise protects against low power visible laser radiation, thus does not function.
- Additional hazards are skin burns, fire, or the generation of toxic products.
- If the laser beam hits the endotracheal tube, the tube can ignite. Combustion of the endotracheal tube threatens the patient's life.
- Laser radiation is dangerously reflected by shiny metallic surfaces.

In order to reduce the hazards to a minimum, certain safety measures should be adhered to. Further measures may become necessary under special circumstances. A surgical laser should be placed in a closed room with a controlled entrance. Laser safety signs and labels should be posted at the doorway to the operating room. Additional warning lights can be used. A laser safety officer should be appointed. He or she should have the necessary technical knowledge and should have received special training pertaining to laser safety. This can, for instance, be the responsible physician or, alternatively, a member of the technical staff of the hospital. Safety education for the laser in use should be given to all personnel in contact with lasers and the respective training should be repeated yearly. Precautions should be taken against toxic fumes or fires. Personal protective eye wear should be worn by all personnel when the laser is in operation. The eyes of the patient should be shielded.

The following *rules* reduce the potential for accidents. They should become habit.

- Never directly stare into the laser beam, even when wearing eye protection.
- Make sure that all personnel are wearing laser protective glasses.
- Never direct the laser beam in any other direction than onto the operative field.
- Leave the laser switched off until treatment is started. Switch it off immediately after the treatment has been finished.
- Avoid the danger of confusing the foot switches.
- Use the stand-by function during treatment pauses.
- Keep the laser beam away from easily flammable materials.
- Protect the tissue areas which should not be exposed to the laser beam with inflammable or well-moistened towels or swabs. Do not use metallic parts as shields.
- Avoid introducing reflecting surfaces into the beam path.

7 Outlook

New developments, trials, and experimental approaches are continually being tested in clinical settings. Authors are forced to restrict the information to the state at the time of publication. In this manual of operative laser surgery the described methods are based on our own experience and long-term results. They have proved to be highly successful in our hands and are assuming a highly significant role in the daily practice of otorhinolaryngology.

Photodynamic therapy, which is not yet a clinically proved form of treatment in the field of otorhinolaryngology, will only be dealt with in this brief outlook on the future.

Aims for the Future

A major goal is the development of the technical and scientific basis for diagnostic laser procedures. Among the priorities of the research activities in Germany that enjoy federal funding, are:
- Optic tomography with pulsed laser radiation in the visible and infrared spectrum (replacing X-rays).
- Development and improvement of systems for laser transmission, i.e., combination with ultrasound (US) or magnetic resonance imaging (MRI) (system integration).
- Further development of the dosimetry of laser therapy.

New Laser Concepts in Medicine

Intensive cooperation between different disciplines is necessary to succeed with the development and application of various new technologies aimed at improving the concept of minimally invasive surgery. This includes new laser generators and appliances which can help to optimize current forms of therapy and open the door for new treatment modalities in the field of otorhinolaryngology.

Improved diagnosis of carcinomas is a field of continuous research. The following goals need to be pursued:
- Visualization of early stages and precancerous lesions in the vicinity of carcinomas;
- Detection of multilocular carcinomatous lesions (carcinoma in situ, microcarcinoma);
- Identification of submucosal tumor extensions (nests of tumor cells);
- Early detection of recurrences:
  - Mucosal changes that are very difficult to detect or entirely escape detection with the eye, endoscope, or microscope;
  - Submucosal lesions or recurrences within scar tissue;
  - Tumor recurrences which appear inconspicuous on endoscopic examination but have progressed away from the lumen toward the outside and infiltrated the soft tissues of the neck.

We expect the following procedures to gain importance in the improved diagnosis of carcinomas of the upper aerodigestive tract:
- *Laser optical diagnostic procedure.* This is also termed fluoroscopy and serves the early intraoperative recognition of tumors. The application of systemic and topical photosensitisers must be further developed with the aim of a laser-aided intraoperative diagnosis of tumor.
- *Sonographic techniques.* The possibilities of US to determine the extent of the tumor externally and through the endoscope must be used to a greater degree. Its role in the early diagnosis of submucosal recurrences must be further developed.
- *Laser technical progress.* Laser systems that are already available must first be evaluated with regard to expanding their clinical use to both more specific and broader applications:
  - *Optimizing cutting characteristics.*
  - *Precise surface treatment.* This can be achieved with the Sharplan switch laser, as it allows the exact setting of the penetration for a given surface.
  - *Interstitial application of the Nd:YAG laser.* In cases of inoperable tumors, this technique can be used to apply the radiation energy within the tumor mass and thereby kill off cancer cells through the heat created.

Photodynamic Laser Therapy (PDT)

The principle of this technique is the activation of a photosensitizing agent by light energy. This causes a photochemically induced destruction of tumor cells. The most common form of this treatment modality involves the systematic administration of hematoporphyrin derivatives followed by a delivery of laser light at 630 nm wavelength.

We have carried out animal studies with hematoporphyrin derivatives and an argon pumped dye laser in continuous wave mode and a pulsed excimer dye laser (Rausch et al., 1993). The possibilities and the limitations of the method became evident in these experiments. One of the most important limiting factors lies in the penetration depth of the applied laser light. Curative treatment of tumors thicker than 5 mm will usually fail. As the infiltration depth of a lesion is naturally unknown before therapy, undertreatment of a tumor with fatal consequences for the patient cannot be excluded.

Clinical applications of photodynamic therapy have shown promising results in the treatment of laryngeal papillomatosis, superficial carcinomas on the vocal fold (Feyh et al., 1994; Biel et al. 1999), and for early lesions in the oral cavity, in the esophagus, and the bronchi. Despite these successes we have not applied PDT in the oral cavity or the larynx due to the excellent alternative in the form of laser microsurgery. This is also partly due to the fact that the ideal photosensitizing substance has not yet been found. The requirements for such a substance are on the one hand selective uptake by tumor tissue with resulting high concentrations and a strong local photosensitizing effect, and on the other hand minimization of the side effect of light sensitization in the skin. A priority of present and future research and development is therefore a maximally specific substance with minimal side effects. The aim is an optimized sensitizer, i.e., carrier system with improved selectivity for the detection of tumor tissue.

At this time CO_2 laser microsurgical excision of early stages of carcinomas is the best alternative. It is an oncologically safe procedure with preservation of func-

tion. The completeness of the resection can be verified by histological examination of the excised specimen. This often implies a combination of diagnosis and therapy during only one microlaryngoscopy under general anesthesia.

New avenues would open up, however, if it became possible to safely remove a glottic carcinoma with deeper infiltration (depth of infiltration more than 5 mm) and to simultaneously preserve the vocal fold by means of PDT. By CO_2 lasermicrosurgery substantial amount of the musculature of the vocal cord must still be sacrificed if a larger glottic carcinoma is treated. Postoperative impairment of vocal function can therefore not be avoided. This disadvantage can only be partially compensated for by successful speech therapy.

A promising future approach might be the *topical application of photosensitizing substances after tumor removal with the CO_2 laser*. The goal is to destroy microscopic tumor rests that might have remained after the CO_2 laser treatment. Delta aminolevulinic acid, a substance naturally occurring in the human body, is particularly suited for this. It is transformed into photophrin IX, which is selectively concentrated in tumor tissue. Experimental studies on animals have been successfully concluded (Davis et al., 1997). Initial clinical trials are actually ongoing.

Literature

Chapters 1–3

Abitbol, J.: Atlas of laser voice surgery. Chapman & Hall Medical, London 1995.

Ambrosch, P.: Laser in der HNO-Heilkunde. Lasermedizin 9 (1993) 153-158.

Ambrosch, P., Brinck, U., Fischer, G., Steiner, W.: Spezielle Aspekte der histopathologischen Diagnostik bei der Lasermikrochirurgie von Karzinomen des oberen Aerodigestivtraktes. Laryngo-Rhino-Otologie 2 (1994) 78-83.

Ambrosch, P., Kron, M., Fischer, G., Brinck, U.: Micrometastases in carcinoma of the upper aerodigestive tract: detection, risk of metastasizing and prognostic value of depth of invasion. Head Neck 17 (1995) 473-479.

Ambrosch, P., Freudenberg, L., Kron, M., Steiner, W.: Selective neck dissection in the management of squamous cell carcinoma of the upper digestive tract. Eur. Arch. Otorhinolaryngol. 253 (1996) 329-335.

Ambrosch, P., Kron, M., Steiner, W.: Carbon dioxide laser microsurgery for early supraglottic carcinoma. Ann. Otol. Rhinol. Laryngol. 8 (1998) 680-688.

Betka, J., Taudy, M., Kasik, P. u. Mitarb.: Clinical application of the CO_2-laser in head and neck surgery. Cs. Otolaryngol. 42 (1993) 203-217.

Biel, M. A.: Photodynamic therapy in the treatment of neoplastic disease of the larynx. Laryngoscope 104 (1994) 399.

Bigenzahn, W., Hoefler, H.: Minimally invasive laser surgery for the treatment of bilateral vocal cord paralysis. Laryngoscope 106 (1996) 791-793.

Bocca, E., Pignataro, O., Oldini, C., Cappa. C.: Functional neck dissection: An evaluation and review of 843 cases. Laryngoscope 94 (1984) 942-945.

Burian, K., Höfler, H.: Zur mikrochirurgischen Therapie von Stimmbandkarzinomen mit dem CO_2-Laser. Laryngol. Rhinol. 58 (1979) 551.

Burian, K., Höfler, H.: Klinische Erfahrungen mit dem CO_2-Laser in der Otorhinolaryngologie. In: Keiditsch, E., Ascher, P. W., Frank, F. (Hrsg.): Verhandlungsbericht der Dt. Ges. für Lasermedizin e. V., 2. Tagung, Graz. 22.-24. März 1984.

Byers, R. M., Wolf, P. F., Ballantyne, A. J.: Rationale for elective modified neck dissection. Head Neck Surg. 10 (1988) 160-167.

Carruth, J. A. S., Simpson, G. T.: Lasers in otolaryngology. Chapman & Hall, London 1988.

Davidson, T. M., Haghighi, P., Astarita, R., Baird, S., Seagren S.: Mohs for head and neck mucosal cancer: report on 111 patients. Laryngoscope 98 (1988) 1078-1083.

Davis, R. K. (ed.): Lasers in otolaryngology – head and neck surgery. Saunders, Philadelphia 1990.

Davis, R. K., Straight, R., Sun, Y.: Intraoperative phototherapy: a comparative study of intravenous and topical photofrin II and aminolevulinic acid. Otolaryngol. Head Neck Surg. 116/2 (1997) 223-227.

Eckel, H. E., Thumfart, W. F.: Laser surgery for the treatment of larynx carcinomas: indications, techniques, and preliminary results. Ann. Otol. Rhinol. Laryngol. 101 (1992) 113-118.

Feyh, J.: Photodynamic treatment for cancers of the head and neck. J. Photochem. Photobiol. 86 (1996) 175-177.

Fried, M. P.: Lasers in clinical otolaryngology: Current uses and future applications. Ear Nose Throat J. 70 (1991) 843-847.

Friedrich, G.: Endolaryngeal laser surgery and stenting for laryngeal stenoses. Kongressband: 2nd International Symposium on Laryngeal and Tracheal Reconstruction, May 22-26, 1996, Monte Carlo (Abstract No 72).

Gandour-Edwards, R. F., Donald, P. J., Wiese, D. A.: Accurancy of intraoperative frozen section diagnosis in head and neck surgery: experience at a university medical center. Head Neck 15 (1993) 33-38.

Glanz, H. K.: Carcinoma of the larynx. In: Pfalz, C. R. (ed.): New aspects of fundamental problems in laryngology and otology. Advances in Oto-Rhino-Laryngology, Vol. 32. Karger, Basel 1984 (pp. 1-123).

Glanz, H.: Pathomorphological aspects of transoral resection of hypopharyngeal carcinoma with preservation of the Larynx. Laryngo.-Rhino.-Otologie 78 (1999) 654-662.

Grossenbacher, R.: Laser in der Otorhinolaryngologie. Thieme, Stuttgart 1985.

Hirano, M., Kurita, S., Shik Cho, J., Tanaka, H.: Computed tomography in determining laryngeal involvement of hypopharyngeal carcinoma. Ann. Otol. Rhinol. Laryngol. 97/5 (1988) 476-482.

Jäckel, M., Steiner, W.: Ear, nose and throat techniques in endoluminal surgery. Min. Invas. Ther. & Allied Technol. 7/1 (1998) 9-14.

Kautzky, M., Steurer, M., Höfler, H., Ehrenberger, K.: Laseranwendungsmöglichkeiten in der Hals-, Nasen-, Ohrenheilkunde. Wien. Klin. Wochenschr. 106 (1994) 45-53.

Kirchner, J. A.: "What have whole organ sections contributed to the treatment of laryngeal cancer?" Ann. Otol. Rhinol. Laryngol. 98 (1989) 661-667.

Kleinsasser, O., Glanz, H.: Histologisch kontrollierte Tumorchirurgie. HNO 32 (1984) 234-236.

Kleinsasser, O. (Hrsg.): Tumoren des Larynx und Hypopharynx. Thieme, Stuttgart 1987.

Kleinsasser, O., Glanz, H., Kimmich, T.: Endoscopic surgery of vocal cord cancers. HNO 36 (1988) 412-416.

Krespi, Y. P., Meltzer, C. J.: Laser surgery for vocal cord carcinoma involving the anterior commissure. Ann. Otol. Rhinol. Laryngol. 98 (1989) 105-109.

Lippert, B. M., Folz B. J., Gottschlich, S., Werner, J. A.: Microendoscopic treatment of the hypopharyngeal diverticulum with the CO_2-laser. Lasers Surg. Med. 20 (1997) 394-401.

Manni, J. J., v.d. Hoogen, F. J. A.: Supraomohyoid neck dissection with frozen section biopsy as a staging procedure in the clinically node-negative neck in carcinoma of the oral cavity. Am. H. Surg. 162 (1991) 373-376.

Medina, J. E., Byers, R. M.: Supraomohyoid neck dissection: Rationale, indications, and surgical technique. Head Neck Surg. 11 (1989) 111-122.

Michaels, L., Gregor, R. T.: Examination of the Larynx in the Histopathology Laboratory. J. Clin. Path. 33 (1980) 705-710.

Pearson, B. W.: Minimally-Invasive Transoral Resection Of Head And Neck Cancers. http://www.dcmsonline.org/jax-medicine/1998journals/february98/transoral.htm

Pellitteri, P. K., Robbins, K. T., Neumann, T.: Expanded application of selective neck dissection with regards to nodal status. Head Neck 19 (1997) 260-265.

Pitman, K. T., Johnson, J. T., Myers, E. N.: Effectiveness of selective neck dissection for management of the clinically negative neck. Arch. Otolaryngol. Head Neck Surg. 123 (1997) 917-922.

Radu, A., Grosjean, P., Fontolliet, Ch., Wagniers, G., Woodtli, A., Van den Bergh, H., Monnier, Ph.: Photodynamic therapy for 101 early cancers of the upper aerodigestive tract, the esophagus, and the bronchi: A single-institution experience. Diagnostic and Therapeutic Endoscopy 5 (1999) 145-154.

Rausch, P. C., Rolfs, F., Winkler, M. R., Kottysch, A., Schauer, A., Steiner, W.: Pulsed versus continuous wave excitation mechanisms in photodynamic therapy of differently graded squamous cell carcinomas in tumor-implanted nude mice. Eur. Arch. Oto-Rhino-Laryngol. 250 (1993) 82-87.

Robbins, K. T., Medina, J. E., Wolfe, G. T., Levine P. A., Sessions, R. B., Pruet, C. W.: Standardizing neck dissection terminology. Official report of the Academy's Committee for Head and Neck Surgery and Oncology. Arch. Otolaryngol. Head Neck Surg. 117 (1991) 601-605.

Rudert, H., Werner, J. A. (Hrsg.): Lasers in otorhinolaryngology, and in head and neck surgery. Karger, Basel 1995.

Scherer, H., Fuhrer, A., Hopf, J. u. Mitarb.: Derzeitiger Stand der Laserchirurgie im Bereich des weichen Gaumens und der angrenzenden Regionen. Laryngo-Rhino-Otol. 73 (1994) 14-20.

Scherer, H., Reichert, K., Schildhauer, S.: Die Laserchirurgie des mittleren Nasenganges bei der rezidivierenden Sinusitis. Laryngo-Rhino-Otol 78 (1999) 50-53.

Spiro, R. H., Gallo, O., Shah, J. P.: Selective jugular node dissection in patients with squamous carcinoma of the larynx or pharynx. Am. J. Surg. 166 (1993) 399-402.

Spriano, G., Piantanida, R., Antonelli, A., Nicolai, P.: Oncological results of functional neck dissection in laryngeal cancer. 1st World Congress on Head and Neck Oncology, Madrid, 1998. Monduzzi Editore S.p.a. (1998) 175-184.

Steiner, W.: Surgical treatment of the cervical lymph node system in laryngeal carcinoma: In: Wigand, M. E., Steiner, W., Stell, P. M. (eds.): Functional partial laryngectomy. Springer, Berlin, Heidelberg, New York, Tokio 1984, 253-264.

Steiner, W.: Endoscopic therapy of early laryngeal cancer. Indications and results. In: Wigand, M. E., Steiner, W., Stell, P. M. (eds.): Functional partial laryngectomy. Springer, Berlin 1984.

Steiner, W.: Endoskopische Chirurgie in den oberen Luft- und Speisewegen des Kindes. Laryngol. Rhinol. 63 (1984) 198.

Steiner, W.: Einsatzmöglichkeiten von Lasern im Bereich des oberen Aero-Digestivtraktes. Laser Med. Surg. 2 (1986) 75-77, 85-87.

Steiner, W., Reck, R., Dühmke, E. (Hrsg.): Funktionserhaltende Therapie des frühen Larynxkarzinoms. Thieme, Stuttgart 1990.

Steiner, W.: Transorale, lasermikrochirurgische Behandlung fortgeschrittener Larynxkarzinome als Alternative zur Laryngektomie. In: Dühmke, E., Steiner, W., Reck, R. (Hrsg.): Funktionserhaltende Therapie des fortgeschrittenen Larynxkarzinoms. Thieme, Stuttgart 1991.

Steiner, W., Aurbach, G., Ambrosch, P.: Minimally invasive therapy in otorhinolaryngology and head and neck surgery. Minimally Invasive Therapy 1 (1991) 57-70.

Steiner, W.: Therapie des Hypopharynxkarzinoms, Teil I-V. HNO 42 (1994).

Steiner, W., Ambrosch, P.: Laserchirurgie des Larynxkarzinoms. In: Roth, S. L. u. Mitarb.: Klinische Onkologie. Sonderdruck der Schweiz. Rundschau für Medizin-Praxis, Bern, 1994.

Steiner, W., Ambrosch, P., Martin, A., Liebmann, F., Kron, M.: Results of transoral laser microsurgery of laryngeal cancer. Proc. of the 3rd European Congr. of the European Fed. of Oto-Rhino-Laryngological Societies „EUFOS", Budapest, Hungary, June 9-14 Monduzzi Editore P.P.a. Bologna, 1996 (pp. 369-375).

Steiner, W., Ambrosch, P.: Laser in der HNO-Heilkunde, Kopf- und Halsbereich. In: Müller, G., Berlien, H.-G. (Hrsg.): Fortschritte in der Lasermedizin 13. Ecomed, Landsberg 1996.

Steiner, W., Ambrosch, P.: Stellenwert der Laserchirurgie bei Tumoren der oberen Luft- und Speisewege. Onkologe 2 (1996) 346-351.

Steiner, W.: Endoskopische Laserchirurgie der oberen Luft- und Speisewege. Schwerpunkt Tumorchirurgie. Unter Mitarbeit von Petra Ambrosch. Georg Thieme Verlag, Stuttgart-New York 1997.

Steiner, W., Ambrosch, P.: Endoscopic Laser Surgery of the Upper Aerodigestive Tract. With Special Emphasis on Tumor Surgery. Georg Thieme Verlag, Stuttgart-New York 2000.

Steiner, W., Ambrosch, P., Hess, C. F., Kron, M.: Organ preservation by transoral laser microsurgery in pyriform sinus carcinoma. Otolaryngol. Head Neck Surg. (in press).

Strong, M. S., Jako, G. J.: Laser surgery in the larynx-early clinical experience with continous CO_2 Laser. Ann. Oto-Rhino-Laryngol. 81 (1972) 791.

Tillman, B.: Farbatlas der Anatomie. Zahnmedizin – Humanmedizin Kopf – Hals – Rumpf. Thieme, Stuttgart 1997.

Van Overbeek, J. J. M.: Meditation on the pathogenesis of hypopharyngeal (Zenker's) diverticulum and a report of endoscopic treatment in 545 patients. Ann. Otol. Rhinol. Laryngol. 103 (1994) 178-185.

Walker, R. P., Grigg-Damberger, M. M., Gospalsami, C.: Uvulopalatopharyngoplasty versus laser-assisted uvulopalatoplasty for the treatment of obstructive sleep apnea. Laryngoscope 107 (1997) 76-82.

Weerda, H., Schlenter, W., Ahrens, K.-H., Bach-Quang, M.: Neues Divertikuloskop zur Schwellendurchtrennung des Zenkerschen Divertikels mit dem CO_2-Laser. Arch. Otorhinolaryngol. Suppl. II (1988) 269-271.

Weisberger, E. C.: Lasers in head and neck surgery. Igaku-Shoin, New York 1991.

Werner, J. A.: Untersuchungen zum Lymph-Gefäßsystem des Aerodigestivtraktes im Kopf-Hals-Bereich. Habilitationsschrift, Universität Kiel 1993.

Wustrow, T. P. U.: Grundlagen immunologischer Vorgänge beim Plattenepithelkarzinom im Kopf-Hals-Bereich – Diagnostik und Ursachen. Eur. Arch. Oto-Rhino-Laryngol. Suppl. I (1995) 221-294.

Zbären P., Egger, Ch.: Growth pattern of pyriform sinus carcinoma. Laryngoscope 107 (1997) 511-518.

Zeitels, St. M., Davis, R. K.: Endoscopic laser management of supraglottic cancer. Am. J. Otolaryngol. 16 (1995) 2-11.

Chapter 4

Blomquist, S., Algotson, L., Karlson, S. E.: Anaesthesia for resection of tumors in the trachea and central bronchi using Nd-YAG-Laser technique. Acta Anaesthesiol. Scand. 34 (1990) 506-510.

Braun, U., Fritz, U.: Die Kehlkopfmaske als Instrument. Anaesthesist 43 (1994) 129-142.

Braun, U., Hempel, V.: Überwachung während der Anaesthesie. In: Doenicke, A. (Hrsg.): Anästhesiologie, 7. Aufl. Springer, Berlin 1995.

Dilkes, M. G., Hill, A. C., McKelvie, P., McNeill, J. M., Monks, P. S., Hollamby, R. G.: The Hayek oscillator: A new method of ventilation in microlaryngeal surgery. Ann. Otol. Rhinol. Layngol. 102 (1993) 455-458.

Grant, R. P., White, S. A., Brand, S. C.: Modified rigid bronchoscope for Nd-YAG laser resection of tracheobronchial obstructing lesions. Anesthesiology 66 (1987) 575-576.

Foth, H. J., Stasche, N., Mungenast, S., Schirra, F. u. Mitarb.: Experimentelle Studien zur Stabilität verschiedener Tubusmaterialien gegen differente Laser. Verhandlungsbericht 1991 der Dt. Ges. für HNO-Heilkunde, Kopf- und Halschirurgie, Teil II, Sitzungsbericht. Eur. Arch. Otorhinolaryngol. Suppl. II (1991) 118–119.

Fried, M. P., Mallampati, S. R., Caminear, D. S.: Comparative analysis of the safety of endotracheal tubes with the KTP laser. Laryngoscope 99 (1989) 748-751.

Hawkins, D. B., Joseph, M. M.: Avoiding a wrapped endotracheal tube in laser laryngeal surgery: Experiences with apneic anesthesia and metal laser-flex endotracheal tubes. Laryngoscope 100 (1990) 1283-1287.

Hirlinger, W. K., Sigg, O., Mehrkens, H. H., Deller, A.: Erfahrungen mit der High-Frequency-Jet-Ventilation bei Eingriffen am Kehlkopf und in der Trachea. Anästhesiol. Intensivther. Notfallmedizin 18 (1983) 243-249.

Hunton, J., Sowal, V. H.: Anaesthesia for carbon dioxide laser laryngeal surgery in infants. Anaesthesia 43 (1988) 394-396.

Jeckstrøm, W., Wawersik, J., Werner, J. A.: Narkosetechnik bei laserchirurgischen Eingriffen im Kehlkopfbereich. HNO 40 (1992) 28-32.

Kurzeja, A., Nordmeyer, U., Weck, L.: Die Anwendung der High-Frequency Jet-Ventilation bei Trachealplastiken. Extracta Otolaryngol. 8 (1986) 66-69.

Mayne, A., Collard, E., Delire, V., Randour, P., Jouken, K., Remacle, M.: Laryngeal laser microsurgery: Airway and anaesthetic management. Hospimedica (Dezember 1991) 32-36.

The Merck Index. 9th ed. Merck & Co., Inc. Rahway N.Y. 1976, 863.

Mushin, W. W., Jones, P. L.: Physics for the anaesthetist. 4th ed. Blackwell Scientific, Oxford 1987.

Ossoff, R. H.: Laser safety in otolaryngology – head and neck surgery: Anesthetic and educational considerations for laryngeal surgery. Laryngoscope 99 (1989) Suppl. 48, 1-26.

Padfield, A., Stamp, J. M.: Anaesthesia for laser surgery. Eur. J. Anaesthesiol. 9 (1992) 353-366.

Perera, E. R., Mallon, J. S.: General anaesthetic management for laser resection of central airway lesions in 85 procedures. Can. J. Anaesth. 34 (1987) 383-387.

Shikowitz, M. J., Abramson, A. L., Liberatore, L.: Endolaryngeal jet ventilation: A 10-year review. Laryngoscope 101 (1991) 455-461.

Sosis, M. B., Dillon, F. X.: Saline filled cuffs help prevent laser-induced polyvinylchloride endotracheal tube fires. Anesth. Analg. 72 (1991) 187-189.

Werner, J. A., Schade, W., Jeckstrøm, W., Lippert, B. M., Godbersen, G. S., Helbig, V., Rudert, H.: Comparison of endotracheal tube safety during carbon dioxide laser surgery: An experimental study. Laser Med. Surg. 6 (1990) 184-189, 197.

White, D. C. (ed.): The laryngeal mask. Europ. J. Anaesthesiol. 1991, Suppl. 4.

Wolf, G. L., Simpson, J. I.: Flammability of endotracheal tubes in oxygen and nitrous oxide enriched atmosphere. Anesthesiology 67 (1987) 236-239.

Chapter 5

Fröhlich, M., Michaelis, D., Strube, H.W., E.: Acoustic voice analysis by means of the hoarseness diagram. I. Speech Lang. Hear. Res. (in press).

Jacoby, P.: Die Doppelventilfunktion des Kehlkopfs und ihre Bedeutung für die Phonation. In: Gundermann, H. (Hrsg.): Aktuelle Probleme der Stimmtherapie. G. Fischer, Stuttgart 1987 (S. 109-115).

Kleinsasser, O., Kruse, E., Schönhärl, E.: Taschenfaltenhyperplasien des Kehlkopfes (Pathogenese und Behandlung). HNO 23 (1975) 29-34.

Kruse, E.: Der Mechanismus der Taschenfaltenstimme. Eine kritische alternative Erwiderung auf die Vorstellungen Réthi's. Folia Phoniat. 33 (1981) 294-313.

Kruse, E.: Systematik der konservativen Stimmtherapie aus phoniatrischer Sicht. In: Böhme, G. (Hrsg.): Therapie der Stimm-, Sprech- und Sprachstörungen, 3. Aufl. Urban und Fischer, München 1988.

Kruse, E.: Disfonia: indicazioni, struttura e metodologia della terapia della voce. In: Schindler, O., Ottaviani, A. (eds.) Stato dell'arte in foniatria e logopedia. Omega Edizioni 1989 (p. 105-109).

Kruse, E.: Funktionale Stimmtherapie – Therapeutisch-konzeptionelle Konsequenz der laryngealen Doppelventilfunktion. Sprache-Stimme-Gehör 15 (1991) 127-134.

Michaelis, D., Strube, H. W. (1995) Empirical study to test the independence of different acoustic voice parameters on a large voice database. Eurospeech '95, Proceedings Vol. 3, pp. 1891-1894.

Michaelis, D., Gramss, T., Strube, H.W.: Glottal to noise excitation ratio – a new measure for describing pathological voices. Acustica/acta acustica 83 (1997) 700-706.

Pressman, J. J.: Sphincters of the larynx. Arch. Otolaryngol. 59 (1954) 221-236.

Rabine, E.: Einige Zusammenhänge zwischen der Doppelventilfunktion des Kehlkopfes und Körperhaltung bzw. -bewegung, Atmung und Stimme. In: Gundermann, H. (Hrsg.): Aktuelle Probleme der Stimmtherapie. G. Fischer, Stuttgart 1987 (S. 219-227).

Rohmert, W. (Hrsg.): Grundzüge des funktionalen Stimmtrainings. Dokumentation Arbeitswissenschaft, Bd. 12 (4. Aufl.). Schmidt, Köln 1987.

Chapter 6

Sliney, D.H., Trokel, S.L., Medical Lasers and Their Safe Use, Springer Verlag, New York, 1993.

Index